The PHYSICK GARDEN

Ancient Cures for Modern Maladies

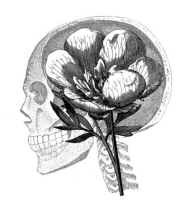

ALICE SMITH

with

Martin Purdy

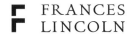

FRANCES LINCOLN

BEWARE

This book contains harmful plants.

CONTENTS

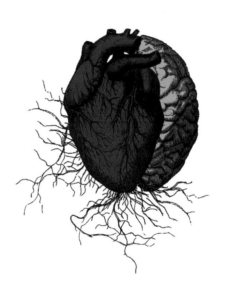

INTRODUCTION

Plants have been used for centuries for their healing powers –
to both positive and deadly effect. Through the ages, these herbal
remedies have become enshrined in folklore, and so too the names
we have given the plants and the old wives' tales we continue to
tell our children. Many have also found their way into
modern medicine cabinets.

This book imagines a physick garden of healing plants
that have been used across the globe by different generations.
But can comfrey really be used to heal broken bones?
And can St John's wort scare away more than bad spirits?
The Physick Garden takes you from the brain to the bowels to
show that sometimes there was method in what
might now be seen as madness.

This book is by no means instructional
and in writing it we aren't recommending treatments.
Neither is it comprehensive – there are notable exceptions.
Our aim is to intrigue, surprise and delight, by offering the curious
and inspiring stories of plants that have historically been used to
heal and of their reappearances in modern medicine cabinets.
It's been estimated by the World Health Organization
that 80 per cent of people worldwide rely on herbal
medicines for some part of their
primary health care.

The illustrations bring each plant to life and hopefully act
as a trigger for your memory, so that next time you are
digging up a root or walking past a patch of nettles,
you will be reminded of the ancient cures
for modern maladies ....

HEAD

brain, nerves, eyes

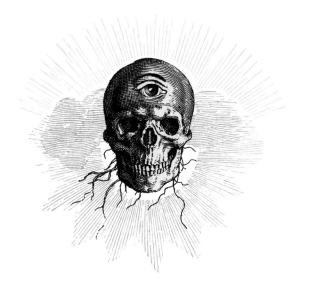

DAISY

Bellis perennis

OTHER COMMON NAMES
day's eye, bruisewort, eye of the day, common daisy, English daisy, barinwort,
lawn daisy, bachelor's buttons, bairnwort, billy button, boneflower,
catposey, shepherd's daisy, dicky daisy, herb Margaret,
March daisy, Margaret's herb

THE HUMBLE DAISY has long been associated with sunlit summer days and the reviving power of sleep, with the term 'as fresh as a daisy' tied to the fact that the flowers close up at night, meaning that they are newly restored on reopening every morning. It is, therefore, not difficult to determine the origins of some of the common names traditionally attached to this hardy perennial, such as day's eye and eye of the day.

Both the small flowers and spoon-shaped leaves of this perennial contain oil and ammoniacal salts reputed to be good for easing muscular pains, but it is the flowers that tend to be favoured more than the leaves. Used throughout the centuries as an ointment for wounds, the surgeons of Ancient Rome would order slaves to pick sacks of daisy flowers so that the juices might be extracted, and bandages were then soaked in them to bind sword and spear cuts. The Roman naturalist and philosopher Pliny the Elder recorded that daisy juices mixed with common wormwood (see page 94) were an excellent treatment for war wounds.

Herbalists and gardeners have used extracts of daisy as a cheap remedy for a range of ailments, from eye problems to eczema, joint complaints to stomach, liver and kidney conditions. In Germany the plant's juices were given as a tonic medicine to stimulate appetite, while the new leaf shoots and flower buds are still eaten in salads around the world.

Research is currently being undertaken into the antibacterial properties of the daisy, but the medicinal values of the plant remain little studied and as such are as unreliable as the chain necklaces fashioned from its flowers.

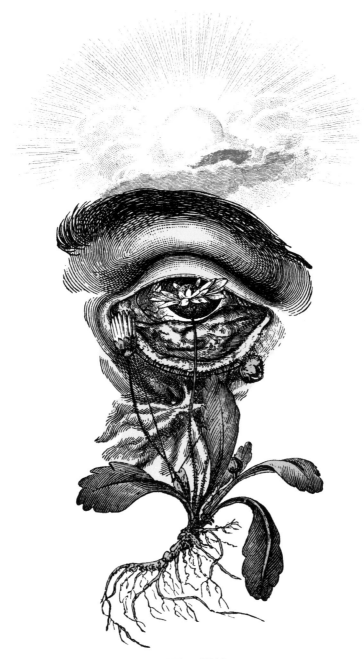

DAISY • HEAD

ST JOHN'S WORT

Hypericum perforatum

OTHER COMMON NAMES
nature's Prozac, scare-devil, *sol terrestris*, tipton weed, grace of God,
devil's flight, balm of the warrior's wound

THIS PLANT IS named after St John the Baptist, and its distinctive, bright yellow flowers secrete a 'blood-like' oil in periods of peak bloom. Such an evocative offering stirred the imagination of pre-Christians as well, who claimed the flowers should be picked before sunrise on what became known as St John's Day (24 June) if protection from evil spirits was to be utilized.

On a more scientific note, research shows that brain chemicals that help regulate our mood (such as serotonin) can be stimulated by the plant, and it is, therefore, often prescribed in tablet form to help with depression, pain and nerve damage. St John's wort is also a popular component of herbal treatments (often in teas, as a tablet or capsule) for mild depression, anxiety, shock and seasonal affective disorder.

It is a short shrubby perennial that is most at home in the kind of growing conditions found in parts of Europe, Asia and North America. Its versatility has seen it associated with bowel and bladder treatments as well as oils for massage and the dressing of burns and sores.

Contrary to popular folklore, modern research suggests that certain properties of St John's wort may have a negative effect on fertility – so any 'married woman' (and, yes, folklore is often discriminatory) intent on following the advice of an old tome, and then going naked to pick the flower on St John's Eve, might want to think of a different way of increasing their chances of conception.

St John's wort is a herb that should be approached with caution, and only after speaking to a doctor, as it can react negatively with a variety of other common medications, including the contraceptive pill. Those who are susceptible to seasonal allergies should avoid this plant, and foragers should not pick the flower in bright sunlight as this can cause rashes. Enthusiasts of folklore might further add that you should avoid stepping on one of these plants unless you want to run the risk of being carried away by a fairy horse.

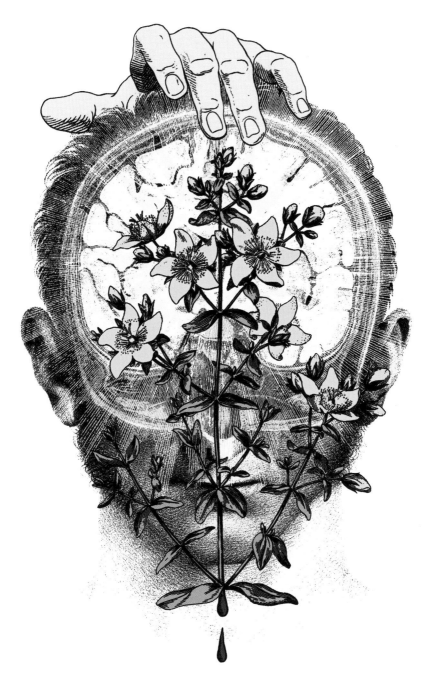

ST JOHN'S WORT • HEAD

CORNFLOWER

Centaurea cyanus

OTHER COMMON NAMES
bluebottle, cyanus, hurtsickle, blue blow, bachelor's buttons,
ragged sailor, corn bluebottle, sultan's flower

THE MEDICINAL HISTORY of this attractive annual is intrinsically tied to the 'true blue' pigment that makes its flowers stand out so vividly in the wild.

Courtesy of the *Doctrine of Signatures* (an Ancient Greek school of thought suggesting that plants that looked like parts of the body might be used to treat ailments of those particular body parts), in the sixteenth and seventeenth centuries the cornflower was prescribed as a treatment for eye problems – its unique colouring was perceived as representing the epitome of what a healthy eye should look like. Cornflower petals are still used by herbalists from mainland Europe in eye-brightening poultices and infusions, as well as in eyewash treatments for conjunctivitis and corneal ulcers. Known to contain lactones, compounds which have mild antibiotic properties, the plant has also been used medicinally as a stimulant to the digestive system, to support the liver and as a salve for rheumatism.

This annual grows 60–90cm (2–3ft) in height and gets its most common name from its ability to thrive in regularly churned-up ground, such as that in a corn field. In France it has become synonymous with the First World War because of the way it proliferated (not unlike the poppy) in the battle-scarred earth. Another common name is hurtsickle, because it would turn the blades of sickles blue during harvesting.

Juice from cornflower petals is used to make a blue ink and pigment that is as popular with watercolour artists as it is with manufacturers of fabric dyes. The petals are edible, which means that they regularly appear as attractive cake decorations – although you might be better sticking to icing for the children's birthday cake as cornflower is also used as a mild laxative for minors.

Cornflower came close to extinction in Britain following the introduction of more lenient chemical weed controls for farmers in the 1970s. Thankfully, a plant that had survived 'the war to end all wars' in the early part of the twentieth century could not be so easily diminished.

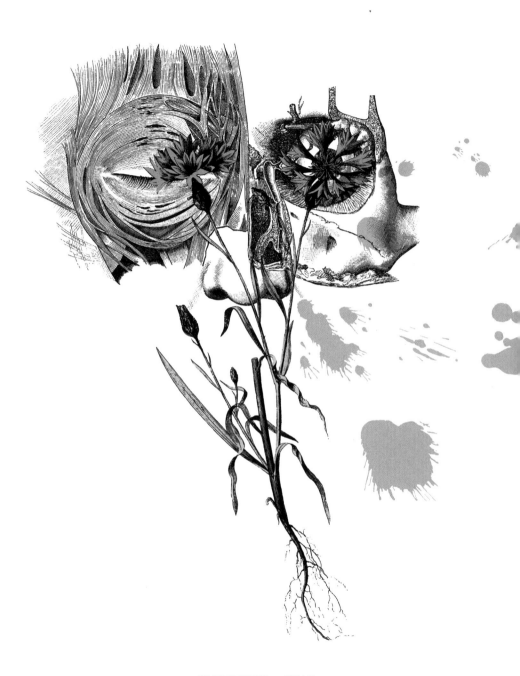

CORNFLOWER • HEAD

VALERIAN

Valeriana officinalis

OTHER COMMON NAMES
Vandal root, sete well, all-heal, blessed herb,
St George's herb, cat's valerian

THE ROOT OF this slow-growing plant has long been valued for its 'anti-hysterical' or calming properties, with the word 'valeriana' even appearing in the eleventh-century Anglo-Saxon equivalent of a modern medical recipe book – a 'leechbook'.

Favoured as a natural and non-addictive alternative to tranquilizers in the battle against insomnia and anxiety, valerian is usually administered in a tincture or in tablet form. To a similar end, valerian tea is regularly drunk as a nightcap in many parts of mainland Europe.

A perennial, valerian develops a long stalk and fern-like leaves and is topped by clusters of small, white and pink flowers. It grows in a variety of soils in Europe, Asia and America and is as versatile in its usage as it is in its geographic outreach. In ancient times valerian was popular with perfume-makers and worn in necklace sprigs by women hoping to attract a lover, although its potent 'leathery' fragrance would generally be deemed too much for modern sensibilities. In fact, the Ancient Greeks referred to it as *phu* because of its disconcerting aroma. The roots of valerian can be used as an aid to those with high blood pressure, epilepsy or in need of support for withdrawal from drugs such as benzodiazepines. Be warned, however, that the smell of a freshly dug-up root may well attract felines (and rats) in your neighbourhood in a similarly hypnotic way to catmint (*Nepeta*), and it seems safe to say that would-be Pied Pipers are likely to enjoy far more rodent-charming success with a pocket full of valerian than an ability to knock out a decent tune on a rustic wind instrument.

An important warning for children: the potency of valerian and its heavy sleep-inducing properties mean it is not suitable for smaller humans.

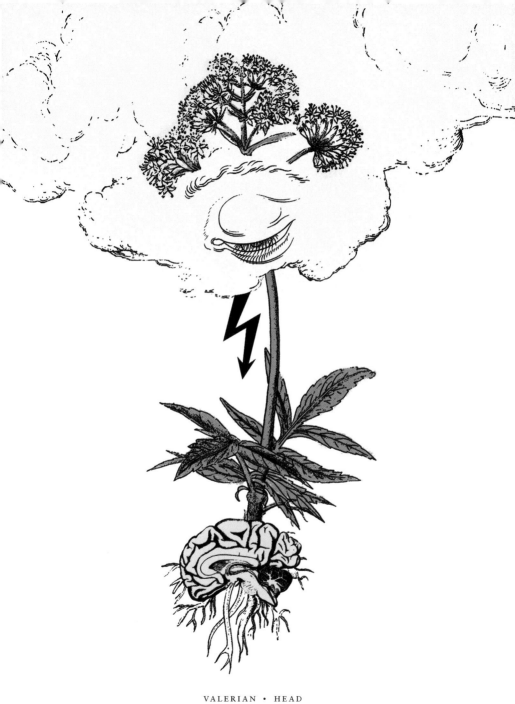

VALERIAN · HEAD

BELLADONNA

Atropa belladonna

OTHER COMMON NAMES
banewort, black cherry, devil's cherry, naughty man's cherry,
devil's herb, dwale, dwayberry

FROM HELPING TO defeat Mark Antony's Roman army in the Parthian war to providing Shakespeare with an evocative weapon of death in both *Macbeth* and *Romeo and Juliet*, belladonna has long held a place in the popular imagination as the 'poison of choice'.

A member of the notorious nightshade family (Solanaceae), this native of Europe, Western Asia and North Africa is undoubtedly one of the most toxic plants in the Eastern hemisphere – but what is less known is that some of its constituent parts continue to be employed for beneficial purposes in conventional medicine.

The juices of this leafy perennial contain the active ingredients atropine and hyoscyamine, which dilate pupils and, in so doing, provide obvious benefits for eye examinations and surgery. Fashionable ladies (particularly in Italy where the word *belladonna* translates to 'beautiful woman') also used to employ the plant's juices, believing that enlarged pupils made them look more doe-eyed and attractive.

Ancient healers would utilize belladonna as a relaxant to ease the pain of distended stomach organs and intestines, as well as a treatment for colic and peptic ulcers. There is some medical foundation for such usage as the plant contains tropane alkaloids that impact on parts of the nervous system that control activities in the stomach, intestines and bladder. The risks, however, are prohibitive – all parts of the plant contain alkaloid poisons, and even imbibing a small dose can result in coma or death.

Thankfully, with its bell-shaped, purple flowers, deep black berries and large green leaves, this is not a difficult plant to identify or avoid. Given its deadly powers, the best course of action is to leave this one in the capable hands of the ophthalmologists – and possibly the witches who, according to folklore, used belladonna to help power their aerial adventures.

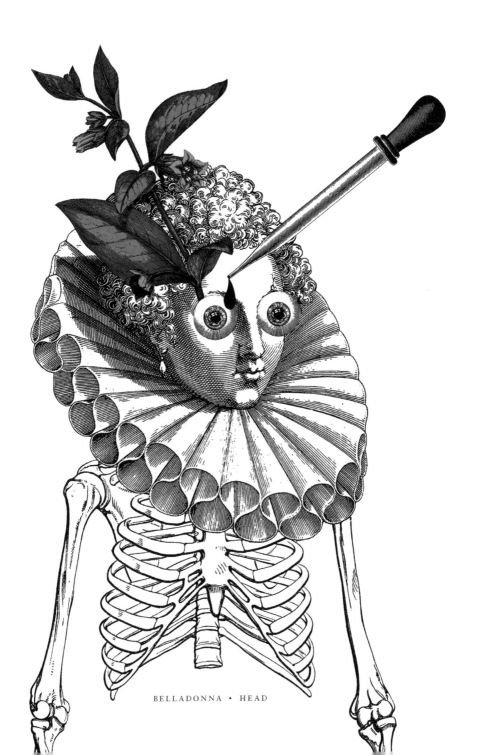

BELLADONNA · HEAD

SKULLCAP

Scutellaria lateriflora

helmet flower, Virginian skullcap, blue skullcap,
mad dog skullcap

NEED TO DE-STRESS? The obvious choice might not be a small flower that bears a striking resemblance to the kind of headwear once favoured by Roman soldiers, but then appearances can be deceptive.

This bushy member of the mint family of North America (whose common European namesake shares similar properties) is a popular herbal aid for the treatment of chronic stress, anxiety, stress-related depression, insomnia and more. It is also occasionally prescribed for epilepsy, withdrawal from tranquilizers and narcotics and to support people with multiple sclerosis, high cholesterol and allergies.

With a preference for open, sunny areas along streams, rivers and ditches, the plant features pairs of attractive, violet-blue flowers that look like small dishes – or like the close-fitting leather skullcaps (*galerum*) once sported by Roman legionaries. In reference to its Latin title, the word *scutella* translates as 'little dish'.

The whole skullcap plant is drawn on by herbalists, although it is the roots and leaves that have always been favoured in traditional Chinese and Native American remedies – these for the treatment of a wide variety of maladies ranging from diarrhoea to chronic pain. Originally used to treat fevers and convulsions in Europe, skullcap is more commonly associated in North America with the treatment of agitation, fear and rabies – the last having been responsible for its popular nom de plume of mad dog skullcap.

Research suggests that skullcap stimulates gamma-aminobutyric acid (GABA), which is a neurotransmitter that acts to calm nerves. It is worth noting that this is also what many anti-anxiety medications seek to do.

Skullcap is widely available as a supplement in capsule, powder or liquid form, and dried parts of the plant (usually the leaves) are also used to make relaxing teas. You might want to consider imbibing such a brew before your next job interview, as herbalists say the great strength of skullcap is that it helps to calm the senses without compromising them.

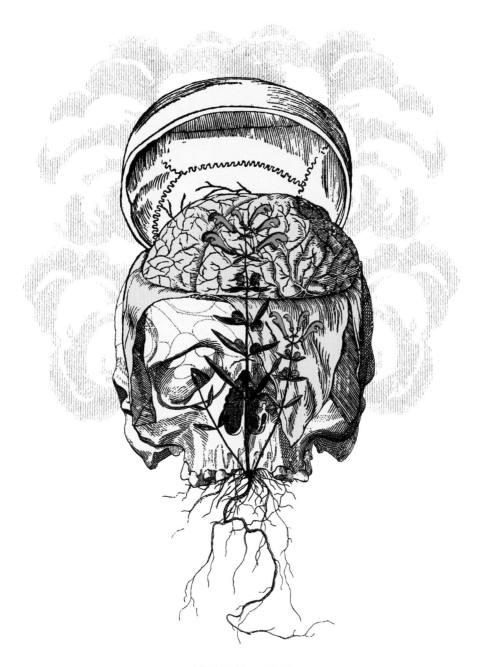

SKULLCAP • HEAD

GERMAN CHAMOMILE

Matricaria chamomilla

THIS LOW-GROWING HERB, with leaves that smell like apples, has been a popular addition to the ingredient bag of natural healers since the days of the pharaohs.

In Ancient Egypt chamomile was revered and dedicated to the sun god Ra because of the way each golden yellow button nestled so perfectly in the centre of profusions of white, daisy-like petals. Traditionally prescribed as a remedy for stress, restlessness, insomnia and associated ailments such as tired and sleepy eyes and heavy eyelids, it continues to be employed to similar ends by modern herbalists.

Flower heads of the plant are usually dried or picked fresh to make infusions such as calming teas, which are also said to have a soothing impact on digestive and gastric complaints. During steam distillation, the flowers produce the aromatic chemical compound chamazulene – an anti-allergen that is useful for treating hay fever, itchy skin conditions, asthma, eczema and allergic eye strains.

Poultices made from chamomile are applied to sore itchy skin, sore nipples and eczema, and clinical trials have proved that the Ancient Romans were right in their belief that the plant has a positive impact on period pains and emotional symptoms such as mood swings.

One of a small number of herbs deemed safe for children, extracts of chamomile are employed as a general soother, while also featuring in a wide range of commercial products for adults, including mouthwash, sunscreen, cosmetics and shampoos.

One of the plant's common names – chamaemelum – comes from Greek and can be translated as 'earth apple' or 'apple of the ground'. It is linked to the aroma emitted by the plant's leaves, but it might also be seen as a fitting description of the way that the plant acts as a 'physician' to its neighbours by nourishing those that are rooted nearby.

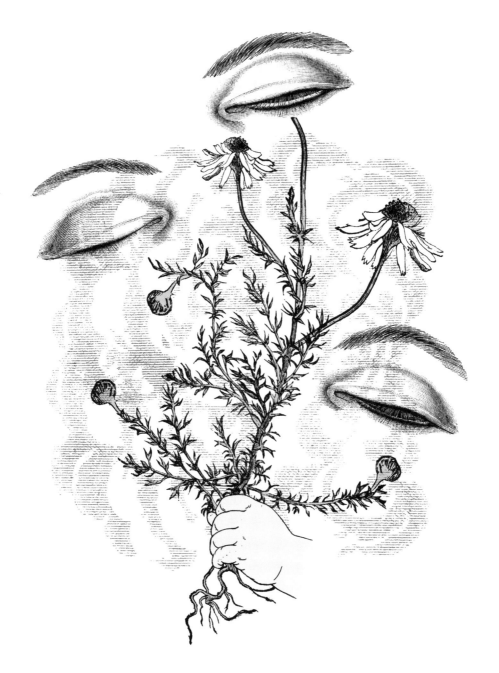

GERMAN CHAMOMILE • HEAD

PASSIONFLOWER

Passiflora incarnata

OTHER COMMON NAMES
maypop, wild passion vine, granadilla

IT WAS SIXTEENTH-CENTURY Spanish soldiers who gave this perennial its evocative title. On arrival in Mexico, the Catholic conquistadors were struck by what they saw as the plant's perfect representation of the Passion of Christ – the flower head's three stigma evoking the nails of the cross, its five sepals the wounds inflicted and its radial elements the crown of thorns.

Extracts from this generally evergreen, tendril climber have been traditionally included in natural treatments (usually in teas) for the reduction of anxiety and insomnia. More recent studies suggest that elements of the plant may boost levels of a naturally occurring chemical in the brain that can lower, or calm, activity in the central nervous system. Research is also well established into exploration of the possibility that extracts of passionflower, which is rich in antioxidants called flavonoids, may aid conditions with links to the oxidation process in our bodies, including Parkinson's and Alzheimer's disease.

A hardy inhabitant of South America and eastern parts of North America, the passionflower is a big fan of sunlight and moist soil and can reach around 6m (20ft) in height. It is something of a favourite with Native American Cherokees, who used the root in infusions for a range of everyday concerns, from the treating of earaches, boils and small wounds to the weaning of children. In much the same way that modern harvesters often use passionflower, the Cherokees also utilized its leaves and summer flowers as key ingredients in a potent anxiety-reducing brew. With its potential to instil a gentle sense of sedative-style drowsiness, airline pilots, long-distance lorry drivers and machine operators might want to give this one a miss.

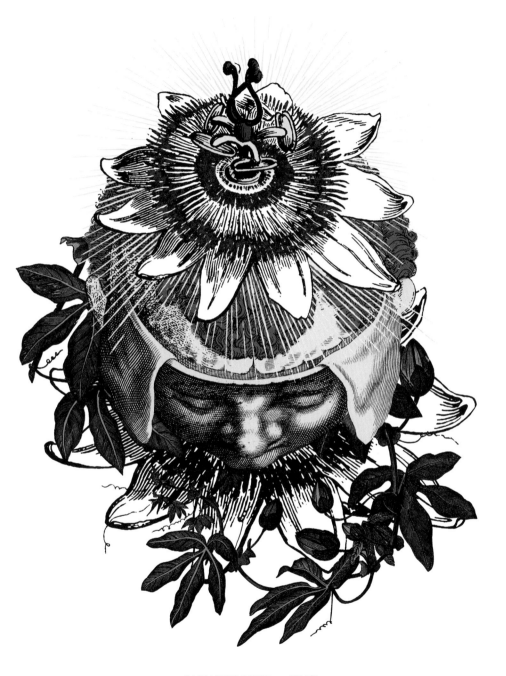

PASSIONFLOWER • HEAD

EYEBRIGHT

Euphrasia officinalis

OTHER COMMON NAMES
red eyebright, euphrasy, eyewort, meadow eyebright

IN JOHN MILTON's epic seventeenth-century poem *Paradise Lost*, the Archangel Michael presents eyebright to Adam in the Garden of Eden so that he can see the world more clearly. It was a reference steeped in history for his readers, and one that continues to resonate today.

Like their ancient predecessors, modern herbalists continue to use this small and elegant annual creeper primarily for the treatment of ophthalmic conditions ranging from redness and swelling of eyes to conjunctivitis, blepharitis and general eye strain. There is evidence that compounds within the herb are anti-inflammatory and antibacterial, making it useful as a counter to catarrh and infectious and allergic conditions that affect the eyes, sinuses and nasal passages. Because eyebright counters liquid mucus, it should, however, be avoided for complaints such as dry eye and stuffy congestion as its astringency might worsen the condition.

Early healers perceived the purple and yellow blotches on the flowers as nature's way of depicting bruised human eyes – resulting in the name eyebright and its appearance in the *Doctrine of Signatures* as a plant to be used for eye conditions.

In addition to its overriding ophthalmic history, it has been suggested at various times that eyebright can also provide further medical solutions: the seventeenth-century herbalist Nicholas Culpeper mentioned that it could be used as a tonic to help improve memory ('weak brain') and it has also been recommended as a treatment for colds and bronchial conditions. Eyebright is common across Europe, where it grows semi-parasitically in grassy meadows and open land.

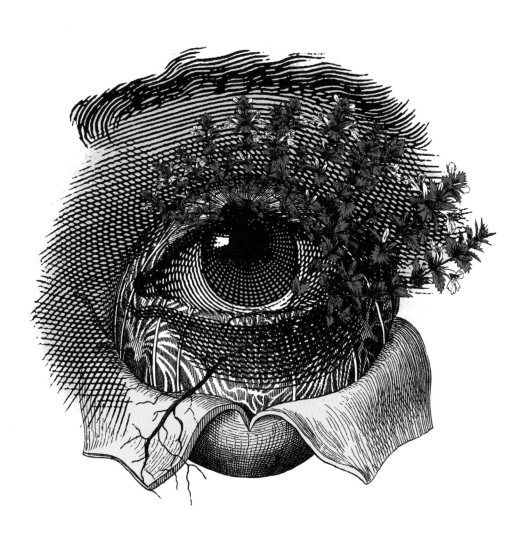

EYEBRIGHT · HEAD

FEVERFEW

Tanacetum parthenium

OTHER COMMON NAMES
parthenium, featherfew, flirtwort, bachelor's buttons,
featherfoil, nosebleed

REGARDED AS THE 'medieval aspirin', the yellowish-green leaves of this naturalized weed have been providing relief from fevers and headaches for centuries.

Feverfew's reputation as a healer has remained strong across the ages, and it has been used since the first century AD to treat inflammations, arthritis, aches, pains and infections. However, it is as a balm for fevers and headaches that it has most commonly served: King Charlemagne, for example, is known to have grown it as a cure for 'fevers of the brain' – and as the ruler of the Franks in the eighth century he must have known a thing or two about 'brain strain'.

Now reputed to help relieve migraines, feverfew is usually taken in tablet form, or else the fresh leaves are eaten on sandwiches to disguise their bitter taste. Studies are ongoing into the impact of feverfew on arthritis, as well as its traditional use as a blood thinner to ease menstrual and labour pains, but the advice of the author of the 1694 tome *The Compleat Herbal of Physical Plants* is beyond reproach. In it, John Pechey told his readers that they should always carry a sprig of feverfew with them when taking a summer stroll as bees and flies absolutely hate it.

A perennial of Europe, Asia and the Americas, this herb's neat and upright flowers are not unlike those of the daisy (see page 8). A regular feature of gardens and waste ground, feverfew can sometimes be spotted in clusters around the rural churchyards of the British Isles – this is because the flowers are said to have been used to provide free floral decoration on the coffins of the peasantry, with some inevitably falling off and taking seed close by. The Latin name of the plant genus (*Tanacetum*) is derived from the Greek word for 'immortal', which may refer to the fact that its flowers can bloom for a long time.

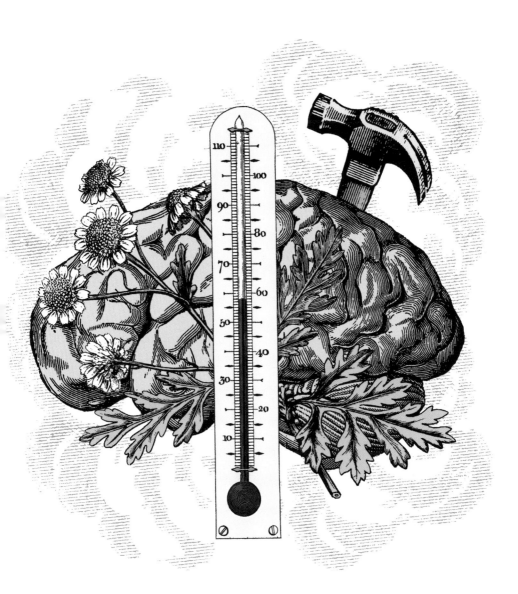

FEVERFEW · HEAD

ROSEMARY

Salvia rosmarinus, syn. *Rosmarinus officinalis*

OTHER COMMON NAMES

old man, rose of the sea, rose of Mary, compass weed, sea dew,
elf leaf, incensier, polar plant, dew of the sea

WHAT'S IN A NAME? Well, rather a lot when it comes to this memory enhancer with its small, needle-like leaves and soft flowering blooms.

Originally a native of Asia and the Mediterranean, where it still grows in abundance on sea cliffs, the species name *rosmarinus* is derived from the Latin words *ros* and *marinus*, which combine as 'dew of the sea'. However, its most common title, the rose of Mary, is tied to Christianity – the claim being that the Virgin Mary threw her blue cloak over a bush and that the flowers were instantly transformed to the same colour as the garment.

Scholars and students in Ancient Greece wore wreaths of rosemary braided into their hair (or garlanded around their necks) to improve their memory during periods of study, and modern research would support them – one of the more consistent contemporary theories being that the herb includes an antioxidant that lowers anxiety levels, so facilitating greater concentration.

Worldwide, sprigs of rosemary have long since been worn in the hair (and combs made of rosemary wood) in the belief that oil from the herb can stimulate blood circulation to the scalp and boost both hair thickness and growth. We can only assume such use would have been frowned on in times of plague, when rosemary was in short supply due to its popularity as a preventative – especially for burning in quarantine rooms to cleanse bad air. Its price is reported to have risen from twelve pence an armful to six shillings for a handful during a plague in England in 1603.

Now readily featured as a food ingredient, as well as in toiletries and bathing products, the popularity of this perennial grows unabated. If rosemary can alleviate even a small number of the ailments it is associated with, from hangovers to bad dreams and indigestion, stress to arthritis and sciatica pain, then we should all be adding it to our window boxes.

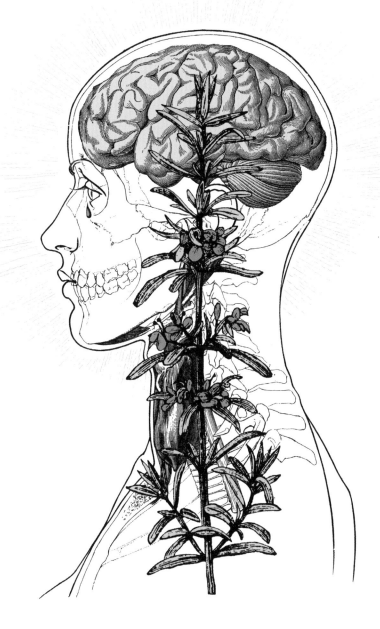

ROSEMARY · HEAD

BILBERRY

Vaccinium myrtillus

OTHER COMMON NAMES
blaeberry, blueberry, whortleberry, urts/hurts, hurtleberry, huckleberry,
myrtleberry, wimberry, whinberry, winberry, fraughan

IT HAS BEEN claimed that the fruit of this deciduous shrub first came to the serious attention of Western physicians during the Second World War, after Royal Air Force (RAF) pilots reported that their night vision improved after they had eaten bilberry jam.

Putting military myths to one side, research has subsequently shown that purple-black bilberry berries do indeed help eyes to adjust to the dark by stimulating the part of the retina most involved in seeing clearly – especially when conditions are dim. Further studies suggest that the berries may also help to improve short-sightedness and repair retinal damage caused by diabetes and high blood pressure.

The power of the bilberry fruit is derived from the number of anthocyanins it contains. Anthocyanins are a type of flavonoid – a class of compounds with antioxidant effects – and are responsible for giving certain fruit and vegetables a red, blue or purple colour. Bilberry's different antioxidants help to preserve tissues within the eyes to reduce age-related stresses, boost circulation to capillaries, improve fluid retention and, quite possibly, reduce the risk of cancers.

The leaves of the shrub may also be used for treating urinary tract problems and irritable bladder conditions and to stimulate activity that can help to prevent diabetes. The small and bell-like bilberry flowers are often prescribed as a mild laxative and reliever of diarrhoea.

Bilberry is usually foraged in moist moorland, woodland and heathland in Asia, Europe and North America. The flowers appear in early summer and the berries in autumn. Across Europe the berries are used for liqueurs, pies and jams.

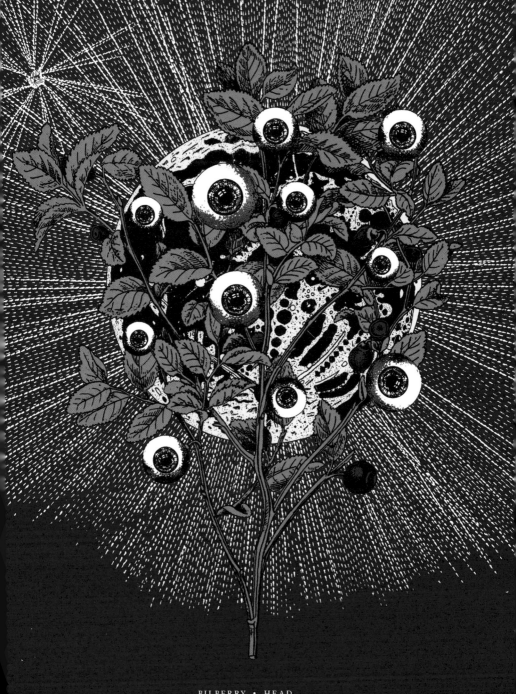

BILBERRY · HEAD

GINKGO

Ginkgo biloba

OTHER COMMON NAMES
maidenhair tree, ancient memory tree

HAVING SURVIVED FOR more than 200 million years, humans
have understandably held a long-standing fascination with the
oldest living tree species in the world – and the secrets it might hold
about the attainment of a long and healthy life.

Popular in Chinese and Japanese temples since ancient times, the name of
this robust tree is thought to originate from a misspelling of the Japanese
name *gin kyo* ('silver apricot'). Its seeds and fan-like leaves have been used
in Chinese medicine for the treatment of asthma, coughs and bladder
problems since the fifteenth century, while it is favoured as a supplement in
the West for those in their middling years who remain keen to 'hang on to
their faculties'.

Having arrived in Europe around 300 years ago, the tree might be said to
be a relatively recent addition to the world beyond its native shores, but few
would have bet against this 'living fossil' surviving just about anywhere. In
1945, when Hiroshima came under atomic attack, six of the trees survived
despite being less than 2 km (1¼ miles) from the epicentre of the blast. Shame
the dinosaurs were unable to pick up any useful tips when they passed
through its timeline.

Ginkgo trees can reach up to 50m (164 ft) in height, and are resistant to
some pest insects, fungus and the most extreme of climates. Its leaves
contain a large level of antioxidant- and anti-inflammatory-generating
molecules known to improve blood flow to the brain. Research suggests that
ginkgo cannot prevent dementia and Alzheimer's disease but may be of
benefit to people already receiving treatment for such illnesses. Likewise,
ongoing studies indicate that it may also have a positive and calming role to
play in supporting the management of schizophrenia, attention deficit
hyperactivity disorder (ADHD) and autism. The fact that ginkgo is known
to aid circulation and blood flow means that it is often taken after a stroke,
and to help relieve the symptoms of premenstrual syndrome.

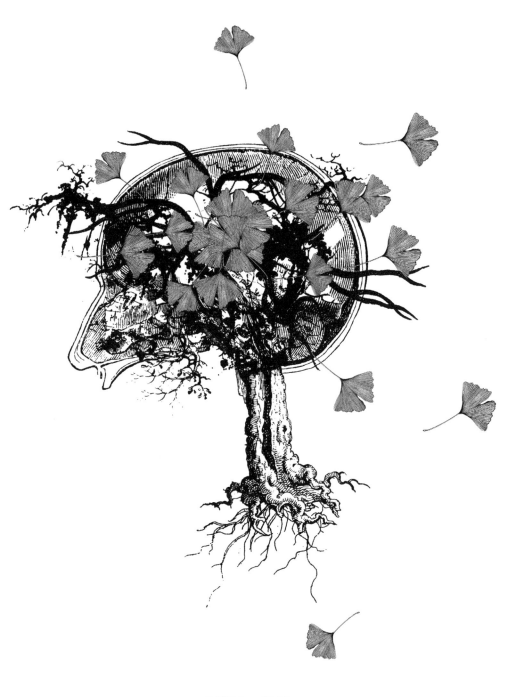

GINKGO • HEAD

CHRYSANTHEMUM

Chrysanthemum x *morifolium*

OTHER COMMON NAMES
ju hua (Chinese), florist's chrysanthemum,
florist's daisy, chrysanth, mum

ALTHOUGH FAVOURED AS a house plant in the West for its ornamental qualities, in China, chrysanthemum is revered as a 'superior' herbal remedy – endorsed by the mythological deity Shennong, and included in the earliest-known Chinese pharmacopoeia, dating back to the first century AD.

Chrysanthemum is a plant that East Asians link to immortality and the slowing down of the ageing process, and is commonly drunk as a refreshing 'tisane' or featured as a 'Ju Hua' infusion to help improve eyesight. The steeped flower heads are particularly popular as a treatment for red sore eyes after long hours of close work involving reading or computing – adherents simply place warm flower heads on their closed eyes and then replace them after a short period with cooler ones.

Chinese healers also believe that this attractive perennial, with its yellow rays of florets, has the power to relieve headaches and counter infections such as flu and colds. In addition, they recommend that the fresh leaves be employed as antiseptic poultices for acne, pimples, boils and sores.

Scientific research has shown that extracts of chrysanthemum may prove of value in treating high blood pressure and angina, while a study by the National Aeronautics and Space Administration (NASA) proved that the plant's reputation as an air purifier is fully justified because it removed a range of potentially harmful chemicals, from benzene to ammonia, from its surroundings.

In Greek, chrysanthemum translates to 'gold', and this humble household staple should clearly be seen as a commodity of high value.

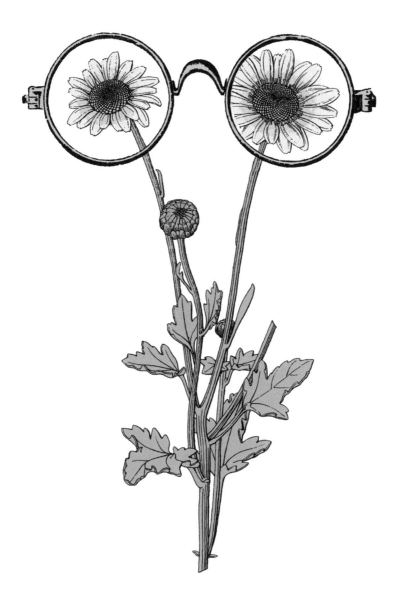

CHRYSANTHEMUM • HEAD

CHEST

heart, blood, lymphs, lungs, throat

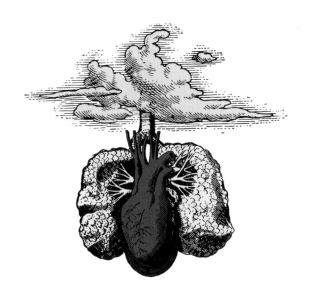

FOXGLOVE

Digitalis purpurea

OTHER COMMON NAMES
fairy gloves, fairy fingers, fairy petticoats, fairy weed, fairy thimbles, witches'
thimbles, witches' gloves, witches' bells, virgin's gloves, Our Lady's glove,
the great herb, fox bells, dead men's bells, floppy dock, dog's fingers,
dog's lugs, cow flop, bloody bells, *foxes glofa*

THE EVOCATIVE AND child-friendly name of this popular staple
of European woodlands and hedgerows makes it hard to imagine
that it was once seen as an herb of the underworld, but there should
be no doubting its toxic power.

Most of us will recall having been told not to touch foxgloves, and for good
reason: ingesting any part of the plant can result in poisoning from deadly
cardiac glycosides – and, as a result of this, early physicians and foragers
tended to avoid the plant.

Change came in the late eighteenth century, when the physician Dr
William Withering went to print with his discovery (unearthed during
treatments for dropsy) that the lance-like leaves of the foxglove had a direct
effect on the human heart. Subsequent scientific experimentation led to the
active ingredients of digitoxin and digoxin being identified and isolated, as
well as the role they have to play in slowing the pulse, increasing the force of
heart contractions and the amount of blood pumped by each heartbeat. The
result? A particularly powerful species of foxglove, *D. lanata*, is cultivated
and harvested on an industrial scale to make heart-strengthening drugs
prescribed globally.

This plant is a favourite of bees, whose visits often help define the tubular
shape of its colourful range of purple, pink and white flowers. Foxgloves
were once referred to as the homes or gloves of the fairy folk, but it is the
earliest known name – the Anglo-Saxon *foxes glofa*, meaning 'glove of the
fox' – that has endured. Linking the two themes, there is an old legend that
the fairies gave the foxes the blossoms to put on their toes when creeping
through hen roosts.

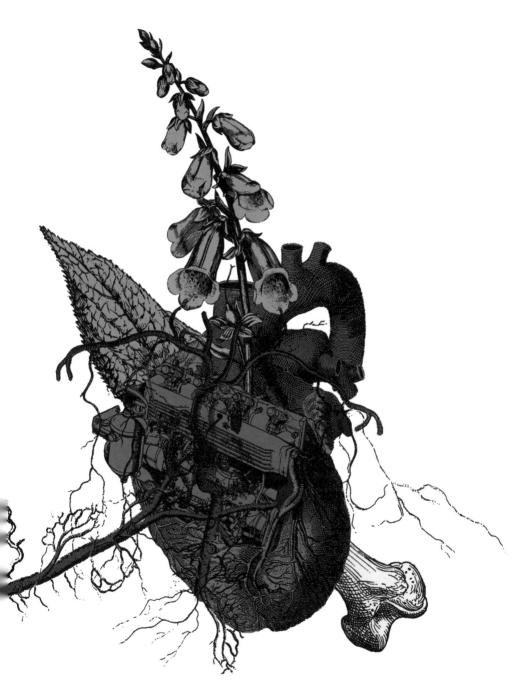

FOXGLOVE • CHEST

ELDER

Sambucus nigra

OTHER COMMON NAMES

black elder, common elder, pipe tree, bore tree, bour tree,
hylder, hylantree, eldrum, ellhorn, Hollunder

ALTHOUGH DEMONIZED BY the Christian Church because of
its association with druids, pagan ritual and magic, the healing
powers of this fast-growing and shrub-like tree are not to be
sneezed at.

Modern herbalists still draw on different parts of elder to support the
immune system against strains of flu, colds and chest conditions, with the
early autumn berries often used for anti-viral impact and the role they can
play in speeding up recovery from respiratory infections. The flowers (best
harvested in early summer) have traditionally been used in teas to treat
fevers, and such infusions remain popular for the soothing of colds and flu,
catarrh, ear infections and irritated mucous linings in the throat and nasal
passages. Extracts from elder may also be prescribed to help lower blood
pressure, act as laxatives and as a support for diabetes.

Given the healing powers of this native of European woodlands,
hedgerows and waste ground, it is easy to see why elder attracted more than
its fair share of superstition. Woodcutters in rural England used to recite a
placatory rhyme to 'Mother Elder' when chopping branches in order to try
and avoid her ire, while the trees were often planted by houses to protect
both the properties and their inhabitants from lightning and evil spirits.
Fans of wizardry should note that wands were often fashioned from elder
wood because of the magical powers that the tree was said to possess.

In a bid to break the spell that the tree had seemingly cast over common
folk, Church authorities claimed that Judas had hung himself from an elder
and that wood from the tree had been used to make crosses for crucifixions.
Such dark and weighty associations achieved only a limited success with
country folk, who continued to make grave crosses from elder wood in the
belief that it could help spirits pass safely over to the 'other side'.

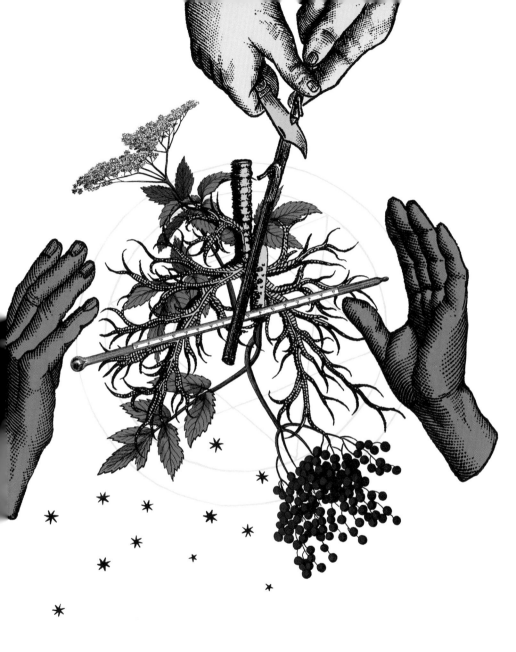

ELDER • CHEST

COLTSFOOT

Tussilago farfara

OTHER COMMON NAMES
horse hoof, horse foot, foal's foot, ass's foot, bull's foot,
hall fort, field hove, coughwort

SMOKING A PLANT shaped like a horse's foot is not a treatment likely to appeal to many, but the bronchial benefits of this tough perennial have stood up to the tests of time.

There are records of the medicinal use of different parts of coltsfoot going back as far as the first century: the Ancient Greeks and Romans are known to have dried its leaves to smoke as a remedy for coughs and asthma, while Chinese herbalists favoured its flowers for use in cough syrups or cigarettes. Coltsfoot is still sometimes smoked as an alternative to tobacco by those trying to wean themselves off nicotine.

Europeans have tended to prefer the use of the leaves or stems of the plant, particularly in herbal brews aimed at clearing congestion, but it was the flowers of coltsfoot that were featured on the signage of Parisian apothecaries as a generic symbol of healing.

Usually found growing on uncultivated land, the small, dandelion-like flowers of coltsfoot appear in early spring and its leaves in summer. The common name of this native of North Asia, America and Europe is synonymous with its resemblance to an equine hoof, but it is the plant's botanical name *Tussilago* (derived from the Latin *tussis*, meaning 'cough') that continues to stir the enthusiasm of herbalists.

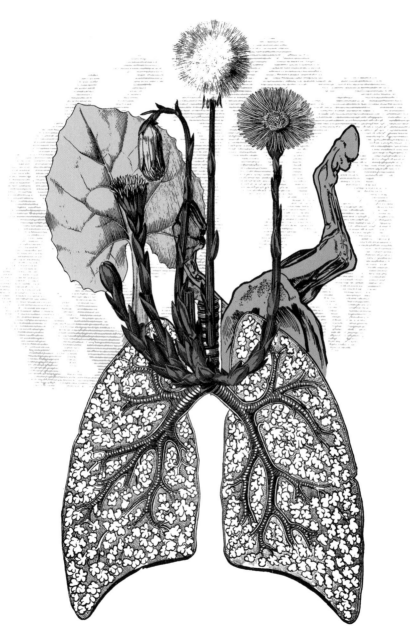

COLTSFOOT • CHEST

HEARTSEASE

Viola tricolor

OTHER COMMON NAMES
wild pansy, field pansy, love-lies-bleeding, herb of trinity, love-in-idleness,
kiss-me-behind-the-garden-gate, kiss-me-quick, monkey's face, three-faces-under-
a-hood, little faces, biddy's eyes, lady's delight, Johnny jump up, tittle-my-fancy,
love in vain, herb constancy, love idol, cull me, cuddle me,
godfathers and godmothers, stepmothers, bird's eye

READING THROUGH THE various popular names of this colourful plant, you could be forgiven for thinking that it first came bursting through the foundations of a music hall or variety theatre – and given that it was the Victorians who did more than most to romanticize it you might have a point.

This ankle-height, short-lived perennial grows in most parts of the world, and its flowers (which come in purple, yellow and white) have generally been perceived as exuding warmth and friendliness and being capable of providing a balm for 'diseases' of the heart. It is for this reason, as much as any melodramatic Victorian belief in its power as a love potion or mender of broken hearts, that its most popular title (heartsease) is likely to have originated.

The plant was traditionally prescribed as a remedy for epilepsy and gout, as well as an anti-inflammatory to treat coughs, asthma, bronchitis and skin disorders. It might also address problems of bed-wetting, 'milk rust', cradle cap and other child-related conditions. There are even suggestions that proteins from the plant may have a positive cytotoxic impact on cancer cells, but research into this remains limited and far from conclusive.

No longer in great demand from modern herbalists, the flowers of heartsease are more likely to appear as decoration on a cake or pricey restaurant meal as a way of providing a touch of 'Victorian fancy'. If you want to impress fellow diners, explain that, according to the Victorians' language of flowers, the purple petals symbolize memory, the white ones loving thoughts and the yellow ones a souvenir of friendship.

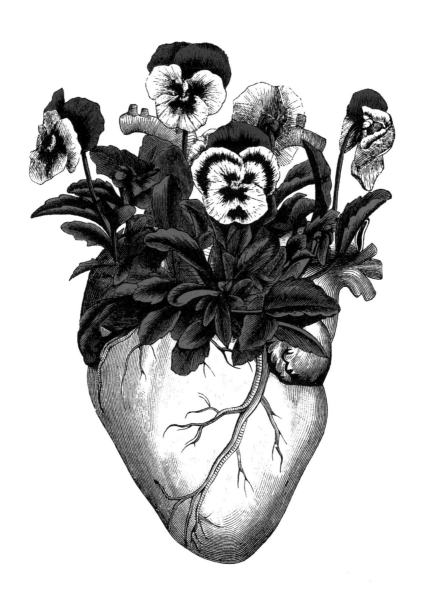

HEARTSEASE · CHEST

KHELLA

Ammi visnaga

OTHER COMMON NAMES
bullwort, false Queen Anne's lace, laceflower, toothpick plant,
toothpick weed, bisnaga

ALTHOUGH THE PLANT traditionally was used to treat wheezing and coughs, mid-twentieth-century researchers developed extracts of this flowering member of the carrot family into a successful support for asthmatics.

This annual can grow up to 1m (39in) in height and is a good source of khellin, a beneficial chemical compound found in the plant's seeds as well as in its soft, feathery and fennel-like leaves. These active botanical properties have since been commercially synthesized for a variety of drugs commonly used to aid respiratory ailments – from allergies and asthma to bronchitis, persistent coughs and whooping cough.

The tall stalk, coupled with the lace-like nature of the plant's flower heads, give it a distinctive appearance, which made khella stand out for ancient healers practising in its natural environs of North Africa, the Middle East and the Mediterranean.

The Ancient Egyptians revered this plant as providing a balm for skin disorders, and the root is said to have been chewed by nomadic North African traders in the belief that it could stimulate skin pigments and offer a natural form of protection from the relentless intensity of the sun's rays. Residents near the Nile delta used extracts of khella as a treatment for parasitic waterborne diseases, such as urinary schistosomiasis, as well as to break down painful kidney stones. On a less dramatic but no less practical basis, the stout flower stalks make wonderful toothpicks.

Modern herbalists recommend eating whole seeds of this species of the *Ammi* genus, or else inhaling the crushed seeds soaked in boiling water through a handkerchief or cloth, to relieve nasal congestion and to combat lingering coughs.

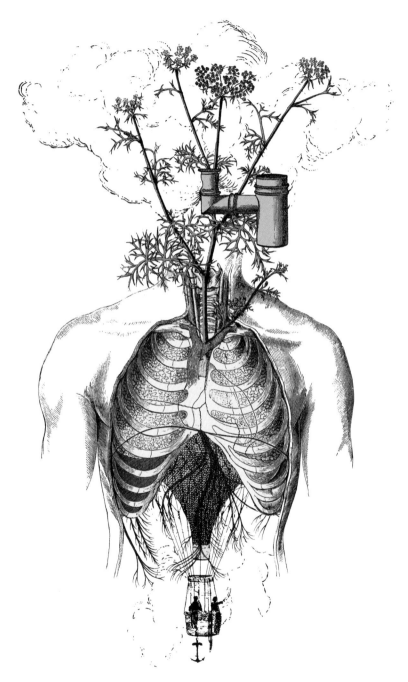

KHELLA • CHEST

HAWTHORN

Crataegus monogyna

OTHER COMMON NAMES
may blossom, mayflower, whitethorn, bread and cheese tree, hagthorn,
red haw, ladies' meat, quick, tree of chastity, pixie pears,
cuckoo's beads, chucky cheese, faerie bush

FROM ITS TRUNK to its leaves, there is little of hawthorn that is not of value, but for those with heart complaints, it is the berries that best support its status as the 'magical tree'.

The tree's berries have been used for heart tonics for more than two millennia. Like their predecessors, modern herbalists use it to combat irregular heartbeats, improve oxygenation and metabolism in the heart, dilate coronary arteries, normalize blood pressure and aid circulatory conditions such as Raynaud's disease. However, one trick that schoolboys used to perform that would help get the heart pumping was to remove the red skin from a hawthorn berry and drop the downy covering of the seed down the back of their victim's shirt – delivering a quick jolt of the 'itchy coos'.

Often grown as a hedgerow shrub, hawthorn leaves can be eaten during fresh growth in spring, when they taste nut-like. The flower petals are sweet and have an almond flavour, but you should not eat the seeds as they contain cyanide bonded with sugar, called amygdalin. In your gut, in the small intestine, this changes to hydrogen cyanide and can have a deadly or toxic poisoning effect. However, the leaves, flowers and berries are all common ingredients in herbal teas, jams, wine and liqueurs.

Hawthorn is said to provide great protection from lightning, and its wood is so hard wearing that it was used for items such as printer's blocks and maypoles. Garlands of blossoms would be hung around maypoles and outside houses to ward off evil spirits and to celebrate the arrival of a new season, new life and fertility. Taking the blossom inside your home was, however, a 'no-no' – a superstition probably linked to the natural 'perfume' of triethylamine released by the decaying blossoms, which happens to be the same chemical odour given off by corpses. To add to this rather macabre imagery, the flowers are mostly fertilized by carrion insects, which enjoy rotting meat.

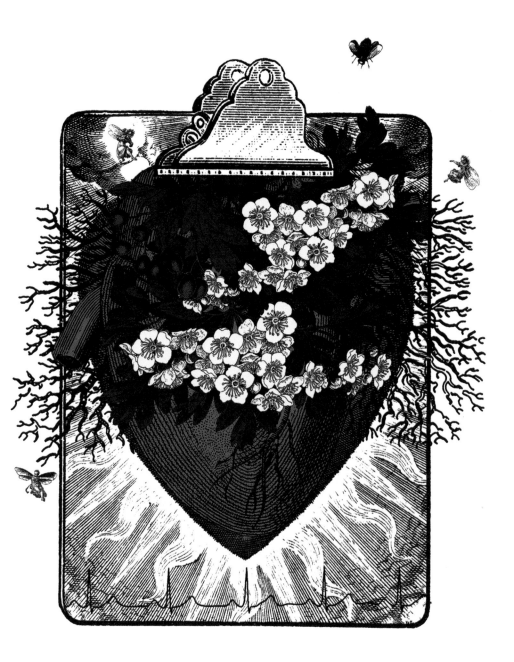

HAWTHORN · CHEST

GARLIC

Allium sativum

OTHER COMMON NAMES
rank rose, stinkweed, camphor of the poor, poor man's treacle,
Italian perfume, halitosis, Bronx vanilla, Russian penicillin, natural antibiotic,
vegetable viagra, plant talisman, rustic's theriac, snake grass

IF ANY ONE plant can lay claim to the title of 'all-round healer', garlic is a contender. With a large body of research advocating properties including more than thirty medicinal compounds (many of benefit to the human heart), it becomes hard to find a bad word to say about this versatile bulb.

Although a probable native of Asia, this plant has been popular in many other parts of the world and the medicinal properties of its bulbs have been so highly valued over the centuries, that clay models of them have been found in the tombs of Ancient Egyptians. Slaves working on the pyramids were sometimes paid in bulbs, which were perceived as a strength-giving 'superfood'. It was also for this reason that Roman soldiers were fed garlic in preparation for war. In twentieth-century conflicts, British medics adopted it as an antiseptic to treat wounds when drugs ran out in battle.

As well as being as an aphrodisiac throughout history, the Ancient Greeks and Indian physicians also used it to treat ailments from seasickness to snake bites and lack of appetite to skin diseases, rheumatism, coughs and more. In times of plague, including the Spanish flu of 1918, necklaces of garlic were worn for protection.

Garlic is proven to help thin blood, to reduce arterial disease and cholesterol, to help with circulatory disorders linked to high blood pressure and low blood-sugar levels, and to increase the potency of antibiotics and anti-inflammatories. In its natural form, it can be eaten raw but, to maximize the benefit of the superfood compound allicin, leave a crushed clove for ten minutes before ingesting it.

Despite garlic's health benefits and the fact that it has been cultivated around the globe for more than six thousand years, the pungency of garlic continues to divide the crowd – with many no doubt sympathetic to the old label of the 'rank rose'.

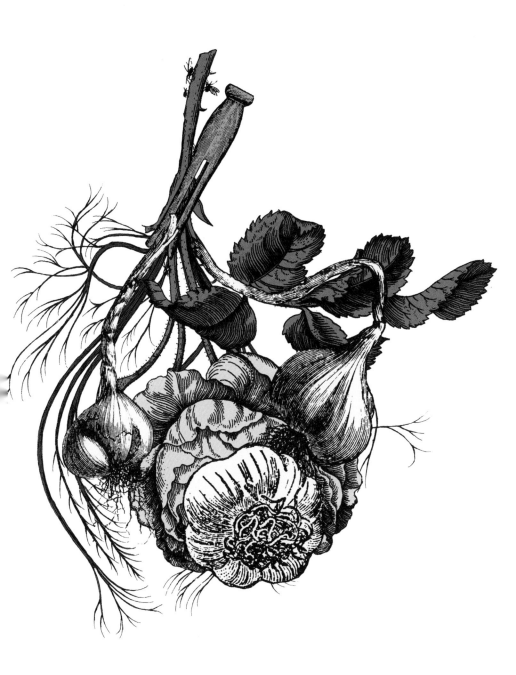

GARLIC • CHEST

LUNGWORT

Pulmonaria officinalis

OTHER COMMON NAMES
Jerusalem cowslip, soldiers and sailors, Joseph and Mary, spotted dog,
spotted comfrey, herb of Mary, Virgin Mary's milk drops,
Bethlehem sage

THE *DOCTRINE OF SIGNATURES* claimed that plants resembling specific parts of the body had been created to treat ailments relating to those same parts, and so the white spots on the dark evergreen leaves of this plant left the physicians of the early Christian era with few doubts – disease of the lungs.

Thankfully, patients prescribed lungwort fared better than most in this highly dangerous pseudo-scientific system because the hairy leaves of lungwort contain silicic acid, which helps to restore elasticity to the lungs and reduce mucilage in the chest and throat.

Dried extracts of the plant remain popular in herbal teas, and it is a common ingredient (sometimes used in combination with coltsfoot – see page 42) of many cough medicines and treatments for wider pulmonary conditions such as chronic bronchitis and asthma.

A native perennial of Europe and the Caucasus, lungwort favours shady damp conditions and produces seasonal blooms that come in both blue and red. Its distinctive leaves tend to be harvested in late spring, and their white spots have triggered a variety of myths that go beyond medical affiliations, including claims that they were formed by the maternal milk of the Virgin Mary or even her, later, tears. Other common names, such as soldiers and sailors and Joseph and Mary, reference the the luminescent blue colour of the flowers.

The influential seventeenth-century herbalist Nicholas Culpeper mistakenly referred to lungwort as the lichen lungmoss (*Lobaria pulmonaria*) in recipes that have gone on to be copied by successive generations of herbalists and druggists. Fortunately this substitution of ingredients has not presented a health risk as lungmoss is also thought to provide benefits for bronchial complaints.

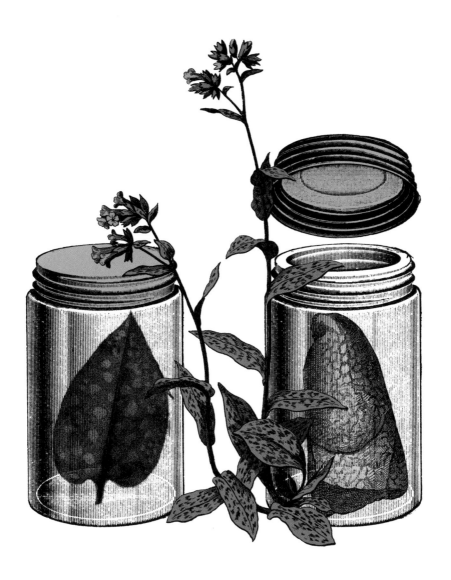

LUNGWORT • CHEST

ECHINACEA

Echinacea purpurea

OTHER COMMON NAMES
purple coneflower, black sampson, hedgehog coneflower, purple daisy,
eastern purple coneflower, Indian head, Kansas snakeroot

FORAGERS HAVE PICKED this native of the sunny central prairies of the USA to a state of wild endangerment, yet its distinctive, daisy-like flower heads and pronounced spiky centres have provided it with a lifeline – as a favourite of domestic gardens.

Native Americans have used this perennial, which grows to around 1m (39 in) in height, for hundreds of years as a cure for a range of ailments from respiratory infections to snake bites.

The flowers and narrow green leaves of three species (*E. angustifolia*, *E. purpurea* and *E. pallida*) are primarily harvested for their medicinal value in summer before the flower cone is fully formed. Patience is required for the more widely favoured roots, which are dug up after four years.

Clinical studies have shown that echinacea increases the number of white blood cells and improves the body's resistance to infections such as colds and flu. Tinctures made from the plant's root are used to alleviate severe infections, while a decoction also from the root can be used as a gargle to treat throat infections and soreness. The juice of the flower head is sometimes prescribed for minor wounds, burns, boils and skin infections.

It is only in recent decades that modern research has confirmed the efficacy of many of these traditional herbal usages, while the specific action echinacea has on the immune function remains the subject of further studies.

The genus name *Echinacea* comes from the Greek word *ekhinos*, which translates to 'sea urchin' or 'hedgehog', in reference to the way the plant's central golden cone becomes increasingly prickly as the flower head matures.

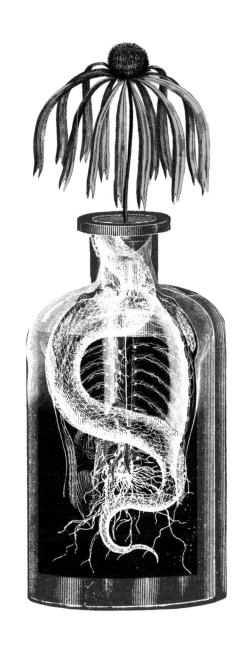

ECHINACEA · CHEST

WHITE HOREHOUND

Marrubium vulgare

OTHER COMMON NAMES
white archangel, hoarhound, marrubio, bull's blood, eye of the star,
seed of Horus, soldier's tea, houndbane, hunan, devil's eye

THIS SOFT AND downy perennial has long been used as a soother of chest complaints, and there is a good chance that the bitter cough sweets or syrup in your medicine cupboard will contain extracts of the plant.

Although known as white horehound, closer inspection shows it is silver in colour (the word 'horehound' is derived from the Anglo-Saxon *har*, which translates as 'grey'). The wrinkly, hairy and nettle-like leaves of the plant, which dispense an aroma not dissimilar to that of musty thyme, add a further distinguishing characteristic.

Traditionally used in brews as an expectorant to loosen mucus, white horehound has subsequently been imbibed in a variety of imaginative ways to similar ends – the Georgians, for example, mixed it in with their snuff, although sucking on a cough drop or candy would unsurprisingly prove a far more popular way to cushion breathing problems such as coughs, asthma, tuberculosis, bronchitis and swollen throat and nasal passages.

Shown to have vasodilative properties – meaning that it dilates blood vessels – women used to be given extracts of the plant to help expel after-births and ease painful menstrual cycles. The plant's proven antibacterial elements have seen it further employed as an antidote to poisons delivered in the form of stings, dog and snake bites and ulcers.

White horehound contains some poisonous elements of its own and can be deployed as a fly killer and to tackle plant diseases like cankerworm, which suggests that it is unwise to eat large amounts in its natural form.

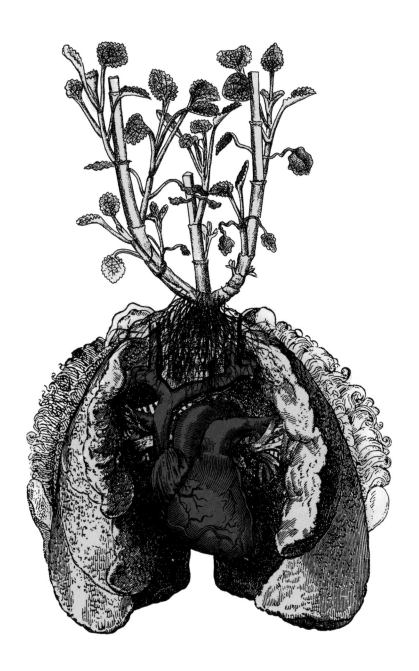

WHITE HOREHOUND · CHEST

BROOM

Cytisus scoparius

OTHER COMMON NAMES
beesom, bizzon, brum, Irish tops, Scotch broom, sweet broom

B E CAREFUL OF making 'sweeping' generalizations when it comes
to this humble shrub, as its cleansing powers are thought to go
way beyond those you would commonly associate with its name.

The long, slender, strong and flexible branches of this European native have
been used for domestic cleaning purposes for centuries, but it is the claim
that its flower tops can act as a form of rhythmic conductor of the human
heart that could be of far greater value.

Many herbalists believe that the plant's bountiful yellow flowers can be
used to help slow and regulate the heartbeat while also combating poor
circulation, low blood pressure and fluid retention. This is a relatively
modern claim and one that comes as an addition to its long-standing and
ongoing use as a form of diuretic and purgative – a practice known to date
back as far as the thirteenth century.

It is worth noting that scientific research into the general medicinal value
of broom remains limited, and that the toxic potency of the plant's blooms
can be highly variable. Clearly, imbibing extracts of this deciduous
plant as a form of remedy is not a step to be taken lightly or without
professional advice.

Mixed messaging? Of course, but we would be breaking with tradition to
provide definitive answers in relation to broom: while twelfth-century
Norman kings were celebrating its deep-rooted tenacity and holding it up
as symbol of noble humility, people in other parts of Europe were living in
fear of using it at the wrong time of year – in parts of Sussex and Suffolk
in England, for example, it was believed that using 'the broom' in May
could see the head of the household 'swept away'.

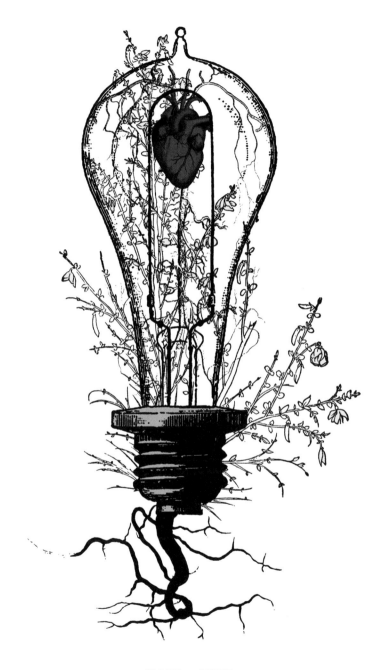

BROOM • CHEST

LOBELIA

Lobelia inflata

OTHER COMMON NAMES
Indian tobacco, puke weed, asthma weed, bladderpod, emetic weed,
gag root, kinnikinnik, low belia, wild tobacco

THIS IMPRESSIVE HERB with potent seed capsules and stem leaves was revered by Native Americans, who believed that the demi-god Wenebojo had gifted it to them after taking it from a mountain giant.

Known as a bringer of good things, Wenebojo lived up to his reputation with this easy-growing annual – it contains the chemical lobeline, which stimulates the respiratory system. Modern herbalists continue to draw on the pulmonary powers of lobelia for disorders such as asthma, pneumonia, whooping cough, pleurisy and bronchitis, and it is not uncommon to see this genus mixed with chilli peppers and proffered as a chest and sinus rub (the chilli increases blood flow to the problem areas relaxed by the lobelia).

Body rubs of lobelia work particularly well because lobeline is absorbed faster when applied externally, and the Native Americans made poultices out of the mashed roots of the plant to treat general aches and pains. They would also rub lobelia leaves on sores, rashes and stiff joints and smoke extracts of the plant to improve breathing – earning it the name Indian tobacco.

In further recognition of the herbal awareness of Native Americans, lobelia is now prescribed for people who are trying to give up the tobacco habit – lobelia has a similar effect on the brain's chemical receptors as nicotine, but without the more harmful, addictive add-ons.

A less attractive pseudonym of lobelia is puke weed, which references its historic use as a form of purgative 'cure all' that could induce vomiting, diarrhoea and sweating. It is for this reason that you are best not ingesting this plant in its natural form without seeking the advice of a qualified herbalist.

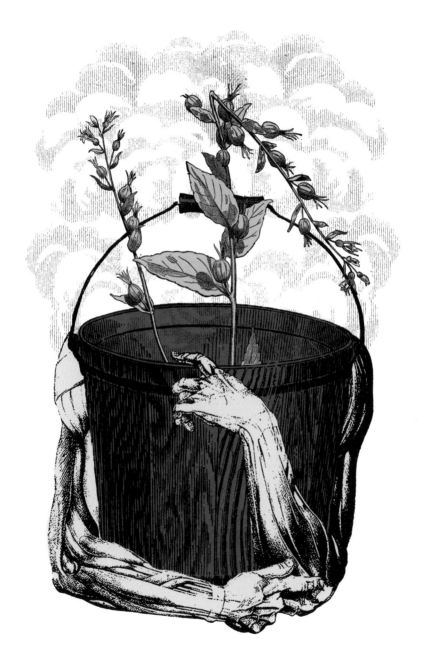

LOBELIA • CHEST

MISTLETOE

Viscum album

OTHER COMMON NAMES
European mistletoe, bird lime, all-heal, druid's herb, druid's weed,
witches' broom, thunder besem, wood of the cross, *Lignum Crucis*,
holy wood, golden bough, devil's fuge, kiss-and-go

THE APPEARANCE OF mistletoe can create some challenging social situations during the festive season, but rest assured that any stress that may result is at odds with the true herbal value of this parasitic bloom.

Found in Europe, America, North Africa and the Himalayas, this plant grows off the branches of a range of trees (including oak, hawthorn, lime, poplar and apple). Its name is derived from the Celtic for 'all-heal', and it has a well-established history as a powerful and magic medicine that is friendly to the human heart.

If using such remedies, it is essential that is taken under supervision and prepared by a qualified herbalist, as mistletoe is a potentially poisonous plant. The dried leafy twigs of mistletoe are used as a form of anti-inflammatory to help lower blood pressure, to ease circulation problems caused by cardiovascular tension and to improve blood-sugar levels and the pathways for nitric oxide – reducing the shrinking of arteries and risk of strokes and other dangerous heart conditions.

The leaves and berries are also helpful in treating nervous disorders such as anxiety, depression and insomnia, as well as a wide variety of respiratory and skin conditions.

The tradition of kissing under the mistletoe is thought to have started in the eighteenth century among the servant classes of Britain, before ultimately catching on with their employers. It was probably linked to ancient fertility rights associated with the plant's ability to thrive and grow on any host partner – a characteristic that led druids to believe that mistletoe had the power to restore fertility among both humans and livestock.

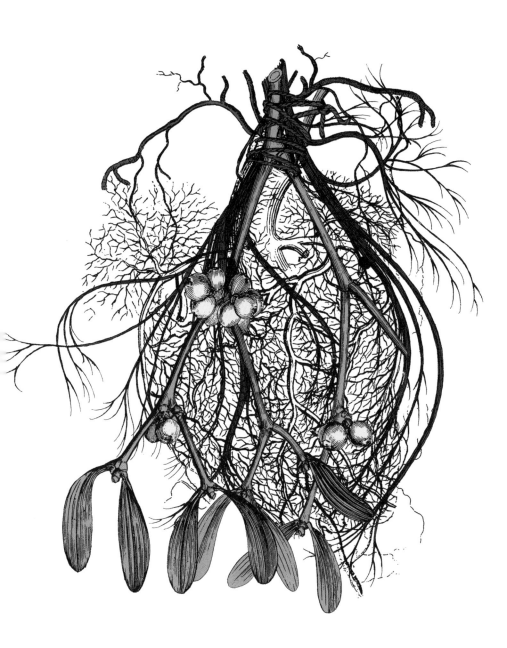

MISTLETOE · CHEST

MARSHMALLOW

Althaea officinalis

OTHER COMMON NAMES
wymote, mallards, mauls, schloss tea, cheeses, althea root,
white mallow, mortification root, Joseph's staff

THIS TALL PLANT, which favours wet, open ground and has velvet-soft stems, comes with a distinct advantage over many of its counterparts – it tastes much better and was imbibed by the ancients for its curative powers.

There are reports that this native of Europe, North Africa and the Middle East was being used as far back as 270 BC as an ingredient in sweet wines. These were popular as cough remedies for the Ancient Greeks. It is also known to have featured regularly in Arabian and Indian medicines.

The Egyptians, Syrians and Romans consumed marshmallow in quantity for its appealing flavour and healing powers, and its leaves and roots remain popular for demulcent qualities that may aid dry coughs, catarrh, asthma, pleurisy and sore throats. The peeled roots (which are rich in vitamins) were given to teething babies as chew sticks, while root infusions were popular in mouthwashes aimed at relieving inflammation.

The generic name *Althaea* is a derivative of the Greek 'to cure', which is hardly surprising given that it has also been prescribed for stomach disorders (excess acid, peptic ulceration and gastritis) and as a mild laxative to aid colitis, diverticulitis and irritable bowel syndrome. The flowers, which are harvested in summer, might have been used to soothe inflamed skin.

Aside from its curative properties, extracts of marshmallow appeared in beauty cosmetics, skin toner and hair treatments – and house-proud Middle Easterners continue to use it on their Persian carpets to help preserve the colour of the vegetable dyes.

If none of this fails to impress, you could simply treat yourself to a sugary confection inspired by a very versatile perennial.

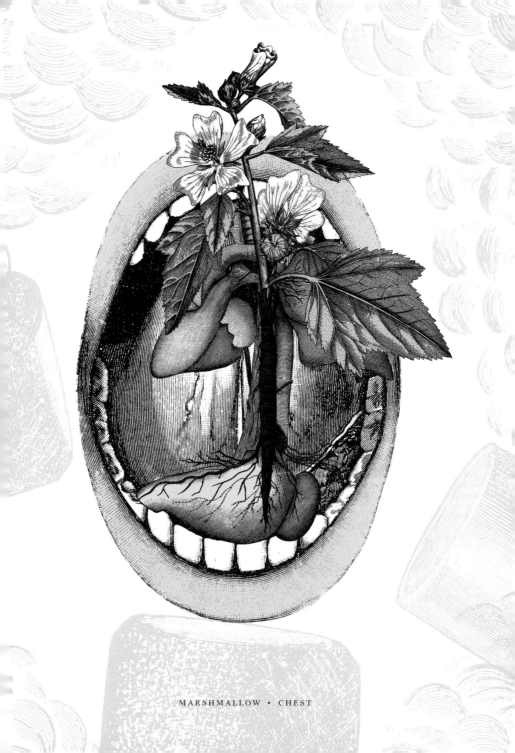

MARSHMALLOW • CHEST

EUCALYPTUS

Eucalyptus globulus

OTHER COMMON NAMES
blue gum, Tasmanian blue gum, fever gum,
fever tree, southern blue gum

HAVING BEEN AROUND for tens of millions of years, this native Australian fire-starter is a true ancient that Aboriginal Australians have drawn on for centuries for its healing powers.

European explorers first came across eucalyptus trees, which can grow up to 60m (200ft) in height, in the seventeenth century. The Dutch seafarer Abel Janszoon Tasman unofficially 'discovered' eucalyptus during a reconnaissance in December 1642; there's a descriptive entry in his journal that refers to a tree that secretes 'gum'. Several decades later, English botanist and naturalist Sir Joseph Banks took part in Captain James Cook's first great voyage across the Atlantic and Pacific Oceans (1768–1771), he collected and recorded thousands of plant specimens and is credited with 'officially' discovering eucalyptus.

Aboriginal Australians use the oily secretions from this prehistoric evergreen as an antiseptic, and surgeons on penal transports are known to have gathered it to treat wounds among prisoners. In 1881 Sir Joseph Lister, a pioneer of antiseptic surgery, supported Aboriginal tradition by advocating the essential oil as a disinfectant for wound dressing.

Modern herbalists continue to use eucalyptus as an antiseptic, but primarily choose it for coughs, sore throats and colds. Sometimes applied as a sinus rub or as an infusion or tincture, it has become such a common ingredient in 'over-the-counter' cold remedies that its smell is indelibly tied for many to memories of childhood 'sick days' wrapped up in bed.

It is believed that an ongoing rise in antibiotic resistance could see plants such as eucalyptus become increasingly invaluable as effective sources of medicine. As the plant has been naturalized across temperate areas of the globe, sustainability should not present a problem. It has become well-adapted to naturally occurring bushfires – eucalyptus plants are known to be pyrophytes, which means they have evolved to be dependent on fires for regeneration and spreading their seed.

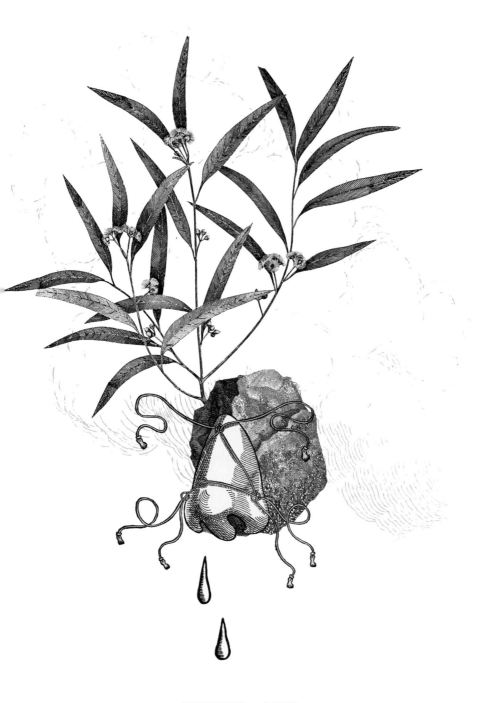

EUCALYPTUS · CHEST

SOUTH AFRICAN GERANIUM

Pelargonium sidoides

OTHER COMMON NAMES
cape geranium, black geranium

NOT TO BE mistaken with your blowsy common geranium, this smaller and more unusual species of pelargonium is a native of South Africa and widely used by Zulu, Basuto, Xhosa and Mfengi traditional healers.

The soft, grey leaves of this plant form a curiously scented and compact rosette around clusters of slightly irregular and dainty, five-petalled, dark red flowers. This distinctive and striking offering is held aloft by wiry stems 15–30cm (6–12in) in height.

As well as being employed traditionally to treat colds, fevers and infections of the respiratory tract (including tuberculosis), it was also administered for dysentery, diarrhoea, hepatic complaints and fatigue. It is recorded that the roots of the plant were used by a tribal healer in 1897 to treat an ailing Englishman, Major Charles Stevens, although it was certainly known to Western physicians long before this – having been first collected by botanists who were part of Captain James Cook's great second voyage of exploration of 1772–5.

Scientific research is ongoing into the full medical efficacy of South African geranium, although that has not stopped extracts appearing in numerous lucrative commercial products as a treatment for bronchitis and pharyngitis. Believed to aid the immune system, the plant is also popular as an herbal remedy for acute respiratory infections such as bronchitis and lesser ailments such as sinusitis and the common cold.

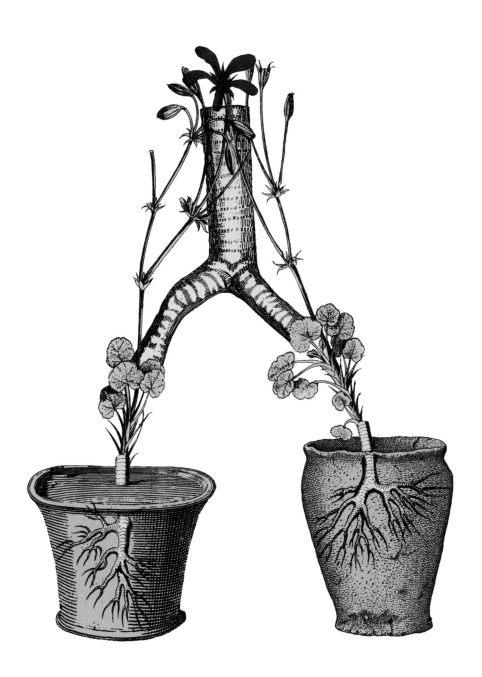

SOUTH AFRICAN GERANIUM • CHEST

MOTHERWORT

Leonurus cardiaca

OTHER COMMON NAMES
heartwort, throw wort, lion's tart, lion's ear,
lion's tail, cow wort

THERE IS A SAYING in English folklore that to drink motherwort is to extend your life to the point of 'continuous astonishment and grief to waiting heirs' – a big claim for a coarse roadside weed.

The regenerative properties of this herbaceous perennial have earned it the title of 'the herb of life', while its Latin name of *cardiaca* references the fact that it has been used since ancient times (in Greece and China) as a treatment for cardiac and heart problems, such as palpitations and rapid heartbeat, as well as a way of strengthening the functions of the heart by promoting blood circulation. Alongside such cardiovascular benefits, motherwort boasts an equally long history as a plant of friendship to females – helping to regulate menstrual cycles and to alleviate contractions and reduce anxiety in childbirth.

The name motherwort underlines the plant's most common associations: female conditions and motherhood as well as the kind of heart palpitations brought on by hysteria. The renowned seventeenth-century herbalist, botanist and physician Nicholas Culpeper concurred with this dual emphasis, writing: 'There is no better herb to drive away melancholy vapours from the heart to strengthen it and make the mind cheerful ... and to settle the wombs of mothers.'

Modern research is a long way from providing endorsements for motherwort's herbal heritage, but it does show motherwort has antioxidant properties that protect cells from damage caused by potentially harmful molecules known as free radicals.

It is the parts of the plant that grow above ground that are harvested and these are primarily used as a tea or tincture for their potential life-enhancing benefits. With distinctive, double-lipped clusters of pink flowers in summer, you will find motherwort growing in woodlands and areas of partial shade in its native Central Asia and Europe, as well as in North America where it is now naturalized (and where it is classed as an invasive weed).

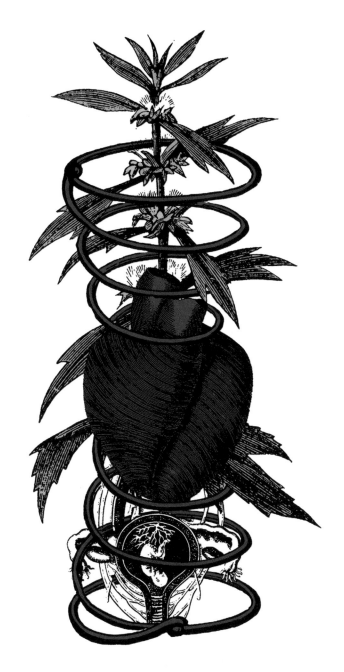

MOTHERWORT • CHEST

SAGE

Salvia officinalis

OTHER COMMON NAMES
common sage, garden sage, kitchen sage, true sage,
culinary sage, broadleaf sage

ALTHOUGH NOW A favourite of the humble kitchen garden, it is hard to imagine that there was once a time when this small shrub was held in such high esteem that those who gathered it would wash their feet in a ceremonial bath before walking the ground on which it had been planted.

Much has clearly changed in the world of botany since ancient Roman times, but if sage is no longer revered as a sacred plant it remains as highly valued by modern herbalists as it was by their predecessors. Primarily it is used as an antibacterial tea to treat coughs, colds and breathing problems; as an infusion to be gargled for relief from sore throats, laryngitis and tonsillitis; and as an expectorant to expel mucus and clear the respiratory tract.

Native to the Mediterranean but now cultivated worldwide, this summer-flowering evergreen thrives in sunlight and well-drained soil, and its velvety leaves (which are best harvested in summer) are pleasantly aromatic.

The Ancient Greeks would bathe in sage infusions because of its healing properties and scent. Roman physicians believed that sage could increase mental capacity, memory and wisdom, and modern scientists continue to research the shrub's ability to address specific problems associated with the ageing process, including memory loss and Alzheimer's disease. In some countries, such as Turkey, they have already found a different way of using sage to keep a more superficial challenge of the passing years at bay – by incorporating it in dyes to darken and disguise greying hair. You cannot deny the wisdom in that.

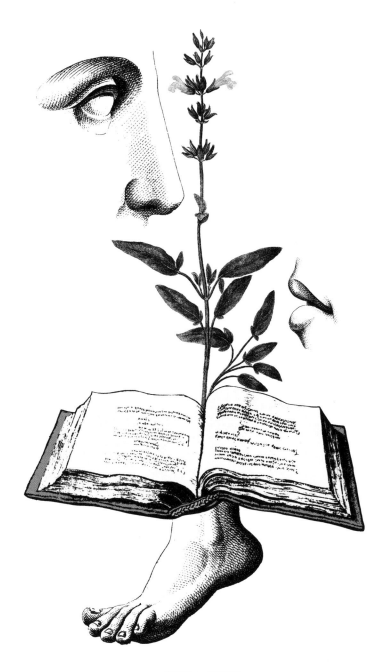

SAGE • CHEST

ABDOMEN

stomach, bowels, liver, kidneys

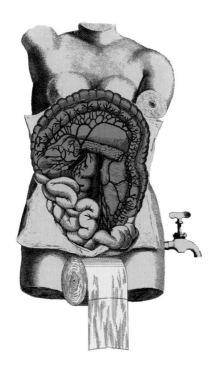

FENNEL

Foeniculum vulgare

OTHER COMMON NAMES
common fennel, sweet fennel, fenkell,
finckle, finkel, Sabbath day posy

EMPLOYED AS A digestive aid since ancient times, modern studies suggest this feathery native of the Mediterranean and the Middle East can relieve intestinal spasms and cramps in a comparable way to a host of well-known commercial products.

The Greek name for fennel was 'marathon', a reflection of the widely held belief that drinking fennel tea has a slimming effect.

The seventeenth-century botanists Nicholas Culpeper and William Coles both recorded fennel as being a dietary aid to 'abate the unwieldiness' of those 'grown fat'. One suggestion was to drink a cup of fennel seed tea before a heavy meal to take the edge off the appetite.

A perennial with a powerful aniseed scent, fennel can grow up to 1.5 m (5 ft) in height and has strong, upright stems with soft, feather-like leaves and yellow umbel flower heads. Now cultivated worldwide, the seeds are gathered in autumn and, like the plant's stalks and leaves, are edible.

The primary use of fennel seeds is to relieve bloating, to settle stomach pain and to act as a diuretic and anti-inflammatory. It is thought they can also help break up kidney stones and play a part in the successful treatment of cystitis. Essential oils and teas made from fennel are recommended as antispasmodics to relieve wind, ease chronic coughs, expel mucus and soothe muscular and rheumatic pain. Further claims are that fennel can reduce bad breath and body odour.

Mild infusions of the plant are sometimes produced as syrups for colic in infants and painful early teething pains. Fennel is also used to increase the production of breast milk. A helpful tip for stable and kennel owners is that fennel repels fleas.

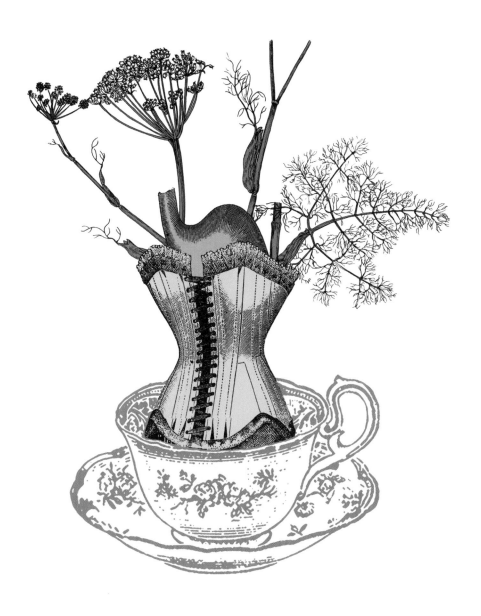

FENNEL · ABDOMEN

ANGELICA

Angelica archangelica

OTHER COMMON NAMES
angelic plant, angelic herb, archangel, Holy Ghost, root of Holy Ghost,
garden angelica, herb of angels, angel's food, holy plant,
St Michael's flower

DIFFERENT CULTURES HAVE deemed this plant capable of delivering everything from long life to a tobacco-style hit, but modern herbalists tend to use it only as a calmer for troubled stomachs.

Angelica has antibacterial and antifungal properties, and the plant's long and fleshy roots are used for digestive tonics and as the basis of concentrated liquors to soothe bronchial conditions, calm nerves (butterflies in the stomach) and stimulate blood circulation in cold winter months.

The stems of the plant tend to feature more in remedies for indigestion and flatulence and (courtesy of angelica's aromatic aniseed odour) as a flavouring for stewed and candied fruit. Its leaves, which are sometimes smoked as an alternative to tobacco in a bid to withdraw from nicotine addiction, can also be stewed into headache-relieving teas, and when crushed and placed in a vehicle are said to calm the stomach and suppress travel sickness.

According to European legend, a monk in the Middle Ages was visited in a dream by the archangel Raphael who revealed that this large-leaved biennial could provide the cure for a plague that was blighting the continent. Whether or not his tip paid off is open to question, but people were still chewing angelica leaves for protection during the Great Plague of London in 1665–6.

If you enjoy vermouth, gin, Bénédictine or Chartreuse, you should raise a glass to angelica when you next have a tipple, as it is a flavouring used in all of them.

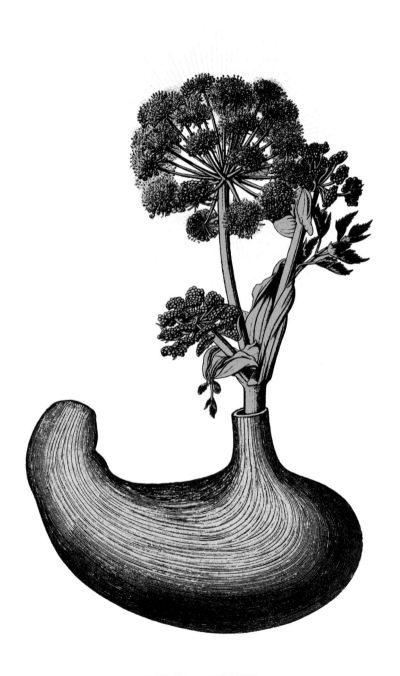

ANGELICA • ABDOMEN

GENTIAN

Gentiana lutea

OTHER COMMON NAMES
great yellow gentian, feldwode, yellow-flowered gentian,
yellow gentian, bitter root

S AID TO BE the most bitter natural substance on earth, this tall and handsome plant continues to be popular with medicinal foragers as a cure for stomach issues and is a key ingredient of traditional aperitifs.

Herbalists, from Culpeper to the modern day, have prescribed gentian as a stimulant for the stomach and as a treatment for symptoms associated with weak digestion, including wind, indigestion and poor appetite. It is also viewed as a stimulant of the gallbladder and liver and is recommended for those suffering from iron deficiencies or for women who suffer from heavy menstrual bleeds.

An essential ingredient of aperitifs like vermouth, such drinks are often served about half an hour before a meal as part of a practice that has always been about more than social niceties: gentian-based drinks stimulate the bitter taste receptors on the tongue, causing it to increase production of saliva and gastric secretions, which in turn stimulates the appetite and improves the overall action of the digestive system, resulting in better absorption of nutrients in food.

This perennial has attractive, star-shaped, yellow flowers and oval leaves, and flourishes at high altitudes; it is native to the Alps and other mountainous parts of Europe, from Spain to the Balkans.

It is named after Gentius, the second-century BC king of Illyria who reputedly discovered the virtues of the plant and gave it to his army to cure them of fever. Gentian was once grown popularly in gardens – a practice that may need to be encouraged once more if the plant is to grow again to a state of natural stability.

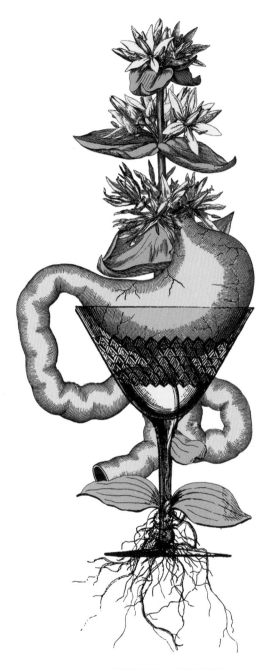

GENTIAN • ABDOMEN

LESSER GALANGAL

Alpinia officinarum

OTHER COMMON NAMES
galangale, galanga, galingale, ginza root,
Laos root, kah, Siamese ginger, Alpina galangal, Thai ginger

LIKE MANY PLANTS in the ginger family, lesser galangal offers a warming and comforting remedy for those troubled by weakened digestive systems. It was introduced to Europe in the ninth century by Arabian physicians.

There are several plants that go by the name of galangal, but *A. officinarum* is the most effective as a digestive remedy. This perennial, which can grow up to 2m (7ft) in height, can be identified by its striking spikes of white flowers with red streaks.

Native to the grasslands of China and South-East Asia, lesser galangal was a common sight on the old trade and spice routes and was purchased by ancient healers to treat a wide range of ailments – from hiccups, dyspepsia, stomach pain and vomiting to diarrhoea, rheumatoid arthritis, seasickness and intermittent fever. It was also claimed that it had powers as an anti-inflammatory, expectorant and nerve tonic.

Offering a pleasantly aromatic and mildly spiced flavouring, infusions to alleviate mouth ulcers and sore gums remain popular, while recent studies indicate that galangal has antibacterial properties that can also help with ear, nose, throat and fungal infections. Higher doses can, however, cause stomach irritations.

Further modern research has suggested that the active compound in the root of the plant, known as galangin, may have a positive future role in boosting male fertility and killing cancerous cells – particularly in the human colon.

The medieval German abbess, healer and mystic Saint Hildegard of Bingen regarded this plant as a 'spice for life' given by God to ward off all ill-health. She wrote: 'And let whoever has heart pain or a weak heart thereupon have a mixture of galangal and wine; the person will be better... let the person who has a burning fever pulverize galangal and drink it with spring water, and the burning fever will go away... let whoever suffers from bad humours in the back or side mix galangal with wine and drink it... the pain will stop.' She may have had a point.

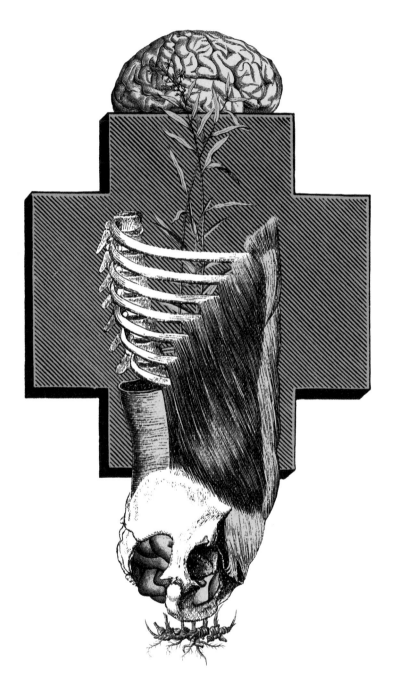

LESSER GALANGAL • ABDOMEN

AGAVE

Agave americana

OTHER COMMON NAMES
century plant, American agave, American century, American aloe,
flowering aloe, Mexican soap plant, maguey

WHILE AGAVE IS mainly cultivated around the world as an ornamental succulent, herbalists continue to value its sap as a remedy for digestive ailments, including infections and inflammatory conditions that affect the stomach and intestines.

Extracted from its succulent leaves, the sap was a key ingredient for Aztec and Mayan healers – and one that would reach a broader readership with the completion of the Badianus Manuscript in 1552 (the first illustrated herbal listing the plants of the New World and their medicinal qualities).

Agave sap was mixed with egg white by native healers to create binding pastes or poultices for wounds, while also using it as a treatment for constipation, jaundice, liver disease, pulmonary tuberculosis and syphilis. Now known to contain beneficial isoflavonoids, alkaloids, coumarin and vitamins, it remains popular as a demulcent and laxative, but it is not to be used during pregnancy or in large doses as it can cause digestive irritation and even liver damage. External application of the sap can cause skin irritations, but this has not stopped generations of males from soaking agave fibres in water for a day before applying it to their scalps – in the hope that it may stop more of their hair from disappearing down the plughole.

A native of the Central American deserts featuring giant, pole-like flower stems and rosettes of sharply toothed leaves, this tall succulent is revered in Mexico as a symbol of abundance: providing food, medicine, fodder, paper, twine, soap, dyes and vital ingredients for alcoholic drinks such as tequila and mescal.

One of agave's most popular names is century plant, which is linked to the mistaken notion that it blooms only once every hundred years, whereas in fact it flowers every eight to ten years before dying.

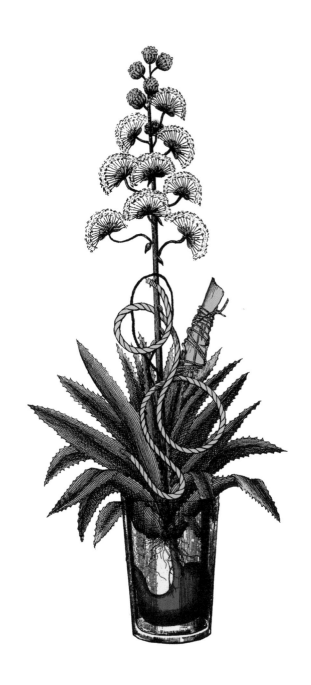

AGAVE • ABDOMEN

GLOBE ARTICHOKE

Cynara scolymus

OTHER COMMON NAMES
heartichoke, cinera, artichocus, globe artichoke,
green artichoke, French artichoke

THIS STATELY LOOKING perennial with its large and thistle-like flower heads has fallen in and out of favour over the centuries, yet it continues to earn respect from medicinal herbalists as a salve for the stomach and liver.

Artichoke's bitter-tasting, 90cm- (36in-) long leaves, with their sword-like serrations and soft, white underbellies, are favoured by healers as stimulants for digestive secretions such as bile, and so are useful for the treatment of gallbladder problems, nausea, indigestion and abdominal distension. The juice of fresh artichoke leaf can be mixed with wine or water as a tonic that is said to protect the liver from toxins and infection, and the herb is also perceived as a useful diuretic for diabetics – significantly lowering both blood-sugar and cholesterol levels.

Native to the Mediterranean region and favoured by the Ancient Greeks and Romans for its edible early green buds, artichoke can grow higher than 1m (39in) and is harvested in early summer. The Ancient Greek physician Dioscorides believed that artichoke had the power to sweeten human relations – recommending the application of its mashed roots to the armpit, or other parts of the body, to soften offensive odours. It fell out of favour in mainland Europe until Catherine de' Medici, the wife of King Henri II of France, reintroduced the plant in the sixteenth century. It was commonly cultivated in monastic gardens, although French women were forbidden to eat it for many years because of its reputation as an aphrodisiac.

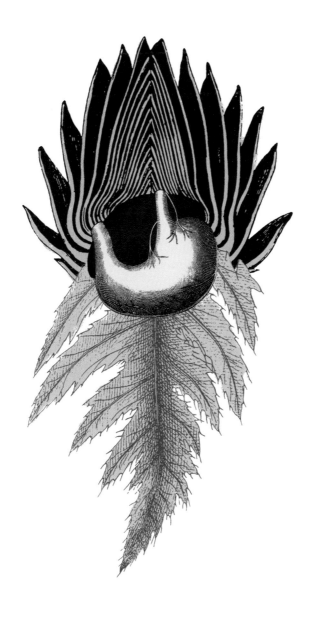

GLOBE ARTICHOKE • ABDOMEN

SWEET FLAG

Acorus calamus

OTHER COMMON NAMES

calamus, grass myrtle, myrtle flag, sea serge, sweet cane, sweet grass,
sweet myrtle, sweet root, sweet rush, sweet sedge

IN WESTERN HERBAL medicine, this lover of wetlands, lakes and rivers is mainly used for digestive problems, although the distinctive, phallic-like appearance of its flower heads has also seen it employed for centuries as an aphrodisiac.

Adherents often chew on a small piece of the root to release some of its juices to relieve stomach bloating, wind, and colic or to aid poor digestive function. The pulp is not to be swallowed – small amounts are thought to reduce stomach acidity while larger doses are believed to increase acid production.

Originating from Asia and North America, this reed-like plant has tall leaves and a creeping, horizontal rhizomatous rootstock. It has been used as an aphrodisiac for more than 2,000 years in India and Egypt, and at Chinese New Year there is a Cantonese tradition of placing the sword-like leaves near the door with a pair of red scrolls underneath bearing the inscription 'Sweet flag, like a sword, destroys a thousand evil influences.'

Taoists believe that sweet flag has the power to bestow immortality, and Mongolians have always planted it near water sources as they believe it helps to provide clean drinking water for horses.

Sweet flag can grow up to 1.5m (5ft) tall and has a spicy, lemon fragrance, which has been used in beer-making and gin-flavouring as well as in perfumes. It does, however, need to be introduced sparingly as the aroma can easily overpower all other fragrances, which probably explains why chewing on the root was seen as providing a quick breath freshener in India.

In some countries, such as the USA, the use of sweet flag is heavily restricted, with the dried rhizome or essential oil seen as being potentially carcinogenic.

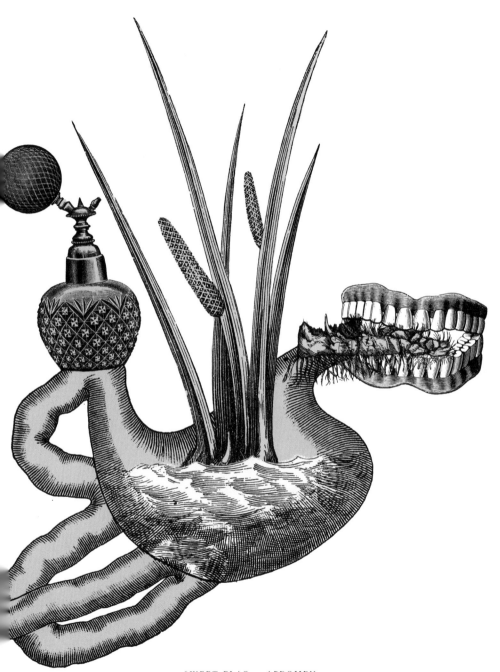

SWEET FLAG · ABDOMEN

MEADOWSWEET

Filipendula ulmaria

OTHER COMMON NAMES

bridewort, queen of the meadow, little queen, lady of the meadow,
dollof, quaker lady, meadow wort, mead sweet, steeplebush

THIS LOVER OF damp places may hold the answer to those nasty
acid indigestion and gastro-reflux complaints that have become
such a staple of modern-day life.

Meadowsweet had an important role to play in the development of aspirin,
with the Swiss pharmacist Johann Pagenstecher discovering in the 1830s
that sap from its stem could be synthesized to create a pain-relieving extract
– one that would turn out to be the same as that identified by the Italian
scientist Raffaele Piria as being present in willow bark (see page 168).
German scientists would subsequently create aspirin from extracts of the
naturally occurring salicylic acid in willow.

Unlike aspirin, which can irritate pre-existing gastric conditions and
cause ulcers, meadowsweet contains a combination of constituents that act
to protect the lining of the stomach and intestines.

Meadowsweet is easily identified by its cloud-like clusters of fluffy, white,
almond-scented flowers. The leaves and blooms can grow to a height of up
to 1.25m (4ft) tall and are best harvested in summer. In medieval times the
fragrant flowers were strewn in church aisles for weddings and festivals as
they were seen as a symbol of love, joy and a happy marriage. This tradition
earned meadowsweet the name of bridewort.

The sweet smell of this herb has also seen it used as a flavouring in mead
and beer and favoured as an aromatic floor covering in earthen houses:
Queen Elizabeth I is said to have had meadowsweet blooms strewn around
her bedchamber for the same sensory reason.

In addition to its ability to calm a troubled stomach, meadowsweet is
also commonly taken as a remedy for rheumatic and arthritic problems,
lumbago and sciatica, while brews made from its aerial elements can help
with headaches, colds and tired eyes.

A genuinely sweet option for any herbalist.

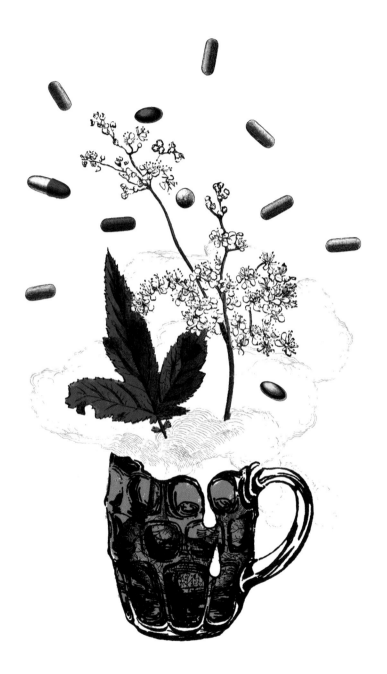

MEADOWSWEET • ABDOMEN

LIQUORICE

Glycyrrhiza glabra

OTHER COMMON NAMES
licorice, sweet root, sweet wood, Spanish root, Spanish liquorice

IN THE THIRTEENTH CENTURY Spanish Dominican monks settled in Yorkshire at Pontefract Friary and cultivated a hardy perennial that would become known locally as Spanish root. They had set in motion a process that would ultimately result in the creation of the famous Pontefract cake, or sweet liquorice.

It is unclear whether the monks or crusading Christian knights in the neighbouring castle should take credit for having first brought this plant with its unfurling, pea-like leaves and small, blue flowers to Britain, but what is known is that it was originally native to South and Eastern Europe and south-western Asia – and it had long since been recognized as a healer.

The Ancient Greeks prescribed the plant for dropsy, asthma, chest problems and mouth ulcers and named it *glycyrrhiza*, meaning 'sweet' and 'root'. In Ancient Egypt it was prescribed for diseases of the lungs, asthma and dry coughs.

A powerful anti-inflammatory, liquorice is still used to treat similar ailments to those identified by the ancients, including Addison's disease. However, it is more commonly associated with digestive problems – reducing stomach secretions while producing a thick lining that combats ailments including gastritis, peptic ulcers, excessive acid problems, irritable bowel syndrome, leaky gut and Crohn's disease. It is also used as a mild laxative.

Japanese research showed that glycyrrhizin, which is one of the key compounds of the plant, is effective for chronic hepatitis and liver cirrhosis, while other health-boosting elements such as isoflavones may help with a range of ailments from eye inflammations to nicotine withdrawal and age-related mental decline.

Such a sweet and extensive medical pedigree for an attractive plant with hidden depths is fitting given that the root system of liquorice can go down to 1.25m (4ft) deep and the stems above the surface can reach to the heavens.

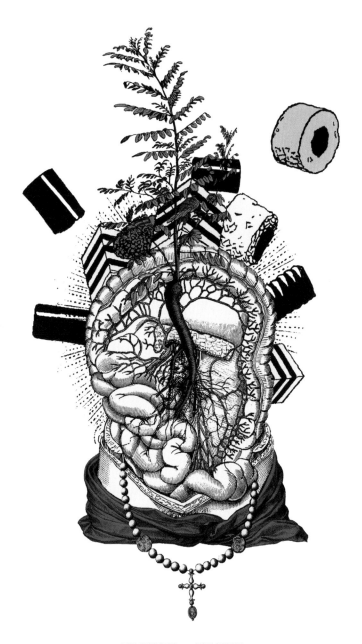

LIQUORICE • ABDOMEN

COMMON WORMWOOD

Artemisia absinthium

OTHER COMMON NAMES
Wormwood, absinthe wormwood, girdle of St John, green ginger,
holy seed, mingwort, old man, crown for a king, warmot

A SK MOST PEOPLE about wormwood and few will get beyond its
role as the main ingredient in absinthe – the mind-bending
alcoholic drink associated with radical 'free-thinkers' like Charles
Baudelaire, Arthur Rimbaud, Pablo Picasso, Vincent van Gogh,
Marcel Proust and Ernest Hemingway. But there is much more to
this musky smelling plant.

A wild-growing native of Europe and Central Asia, Ancient Greek
physician Dioscorides and Ancient Roman Pliny the Elder deemed
common wormwood a stomach tonic fit for emperors like Claudius
and Nero.

Mainly ingested through tincture and teas, extracts of the plant are best
sipped in small doses: modern scientific studies show that its intense and
bitter taste plays an important part in its overall therapeutic power –
affecting the bitter taste receptor on the tongue and setting off a reflex action
that stimulates stomach and other digestive secretions. A drink before meals
can stimulate digestion and improve absorption of nutrients, making it
useful for conditions such as anaemia, while also preventing subsequent
attacks of heartburn or flatulence.

Clinical trials to test the impact of common wormwood on Crohn's
disease have produced some highly positive results. The participants in such
trials also experienced lower levels of depression, which is in keeping with
the use of essential oils of the plant for therapeutic impacts.

Because it is a good insect repellent, bunches of common wormwood are
hung in chicken coops to deter flies, lice and fleas, and it is often prescribed
by herbalists as a treatment for parasitic infections of the gut in both
animals and humans.

If any of the above has helped this aromatic wayside plant to worm its way
into your affections, it is the aerial elements that are deemed as being of
most medicinal benefit.

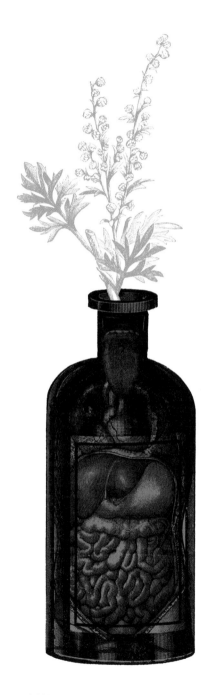

COMMON WORMWOOD · ABDOMEN

GINGER

Zingiber officinale

OTHER COMMON NAMES

common ginger, ginger root, Jamaica ginger, red ginger,
stem ginger, sweet ginger, shunthi, adrak

THIS AROMATIC PLANT was one of the most prized and commonly traded spices during the latter part of the medieval period – a 450g (1lb) weight of ginger root could cost the equivalent of a whole sheep in England in the fourteenth century.

Familiar as a spice and flavouring, ginger is also one of the world's best-known healers. The revered Chinese philosopher and politician Confucius (551–479 BC) was known to have eaten ginger with every meal as a digestive aid and support for flatulence.

Ginger is a rhizomatous perennial that needs subtropical conditions to thrive, and it helps most stomach conditions from indigestion to nausea, excess wind to bloating and cramps. Most impressively, it achieves this whether taken as an infusion, juice, tincture, powder or when eaten as a raw root.

Clinical trials indicate that antiseptic activity within the plant makes it useful for gastrointestinal infections including food poisoning, and that it can also reduce nausea and sickness, including travel and morning sickness. Further modern studies suggest that ginger can also provide a pain-relieving boost for tired and aching muscles, improve iron absorption for people suffering with anaemia and help control fevers.

All things taken into consideration, this rhizome, with its creeping rootstock and underground stem system, has surely shown itself to be worth the price of a medieval sheep.

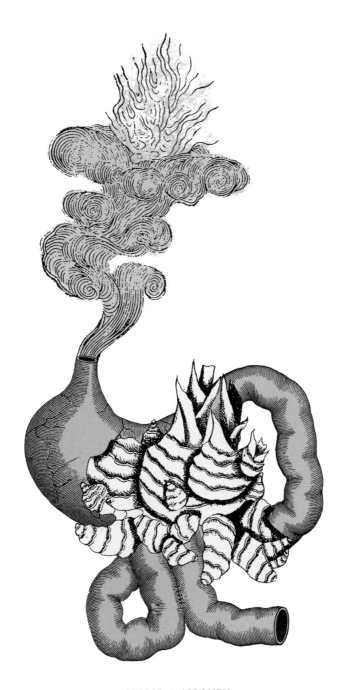

GINGER • ABDOMEN

MILK THISTLE

Silybum marianum

OTHER COMMON NAMES
Our Lady's thistle, Marian thistle, blessed milk thistle,
Mary thistle, Saint Mary's thistle, Mediterranean milk thistle,
variegated thistle, wild artichoke

THE SEEDS OF this prickly thistle have been nurtured as a cure for the liver for thousands of years, and modern research underlines just how remarkable it is in protecting this vital organ from a range of poisons – from alcohol to gallstones, dangerous mushrooms and skin diseases to the hazards of toxic occupational chemicals.

Modern Western herbalists use the seeds to renew liver cells and help protect and treat most conditions that put the liver under stress, including infections, excess alcohol consumption, hepatitis and jaundice. Several clinical trials have shown that the compound silymarin is present in the plant seeds, which can prove effective at protecting liver function during chemotherapy treatment.

In addition to the seeds, the fresh or dried, disc-shaped, white or purple flower heads of milk thistle can be consumed as a form of tonic food when harvested in full bloom. They are generally boiled and eaten like artichokes and were once deemed useful as a spring tonic after the winter months, when our ancestors tended to be deprived of vegetables.

The plant's name is derived from the splashes of white on its glossy green leaves and the milky sap contained within. Early physicians saw a link between the visual and practical and claimed it could help increase breast milk production. John Evelyn – the famous seventeenth-century English diarist and gardener – wrote of the plant's strength as a support for 'nurses' who breastfed the babies of others: 'Disarmed of its prickles and boiled, it is worthy of esteem, and thought to be a great breeder of milk and proper diet for women who are nurses.'

In archaic medical thinking the health of the liver was intrinsically linked with states of depression and melancholia. Now cultivated as an attractive ornamental that can grow up to 1.75m (6ft) tall, milk thistle is certainly capable of lifting the spirits of most domestic gardeners.

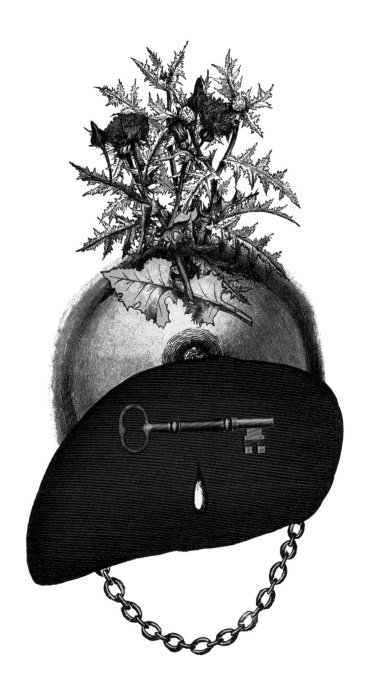

MILK THISTLE • ABDOMEN

PELVIS

reproductive, urinary

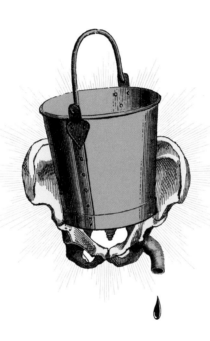

DANDELION

Taraxacum officinale

OTHER COMMON NAMES

dent de lion, lion's tooth, lion's teeth, teeth of lion, swine's snout, cankerwort, blowball, puffball, white endive, wild endive, clockflower, tell-the-time, fairy clock, clock, clocks and watches, farmer's clocks, old man's clock, one clock, priest's crown, pee-in-the-beds, wetweed

THE LEAVES OF THIS powerful diuretic and detoxifier should really be a staple of most salads – being rich in vitamins A, B, C and D and containing a higher count of vitamin A than the more commonly featured carrot.

Modern research has shown the perennial, which comes in more than 1,000 species, can help lower high blood pressure by reducing the volume of fluid in the body. Dandelion can also stimulate the liver and gall bladder to clear waste from the system and so reduce risks of internal infections – a truth that may well provide origins for the old wives' tale that eating dandelion makes you wet the bed.

The root of dandelion is a prebiotic that is typically taken to address constipation, skin problems, eczema and arthritic conditions. It was traditionally used in early stages of late-onset diabetes to stimulate insulin from the pancreas and to stabilize blood-sugar levels, and modern studies suggest that it may have a role to play in battling cancerous tumours.

The name dandelion is translated from the French *dent de lion* ('lion's teeth'), which refers to the deeply serrated and tooth-like leaves and jagged, yellow flower parts of the plant. Such references recur with regularity, with lion's tooth and teeth of lion being just two of its common names.

This plant grows wild in most of Europe and is cultivated in France and Germany, where the leaves are harvested annually in spring and the roots left for two years.

In folklore, dandelion's small and fluffy seed heads were blown to tell the time, how long you had left to live and whether your lover had reservations about your relationship. They can be more usefully used as a barometer: in fine weather, the flower head extends fully and opens right out but shuts like an umbrella when rain is approaching.

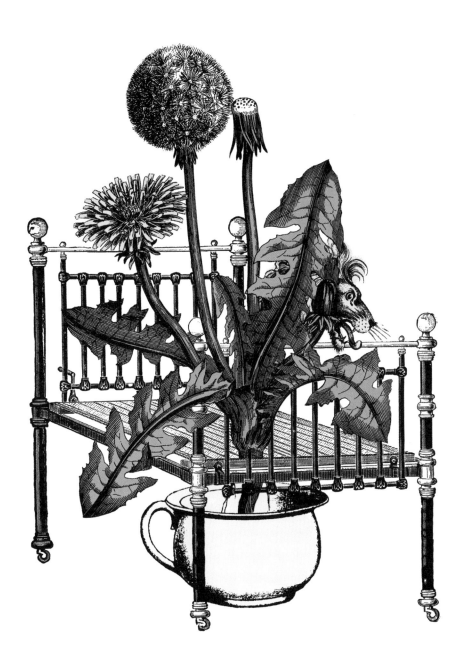

DANDELION • PELVIS

RASPBERRY LEAF

Rubus idaeus

OTHER COMMON NAMES

common raspberry, European raspberry, garden raspberry, framboys,
hindberry, hineberry, red raspberry, wild raspberry

VIEWED AS A friend to pregnant women, the pale green leaves of
wild-growing raspberry have long been recommended by
midwives as a way of hastening childbirth. The chemical actions
that would give scientific credence to the claim remain unclear, but
it is thought the leaves may act to strengthen the longitudinal
muscles of the uterus – so increasing the force of contractions.

It has been suggested that raspberry leaf can promote a quicker and easier
birth, as well as allegedly reducing morning sickness. In spite of this reputation, it should always be avoided during the early stages of pregnancy.

A native of Europe, Asia and North America, the leaves of this deciduous
shrub are harvested in early summer prior to the fruit ripening in high
summer or early autumn. Pickers need to be cautious as the leaves grow on
woody stems with troublesome prickles, and growers also find the plant's
anarchic runner shoots a nuisance.

It is said in Greek folklore that the gods were often found at Mount Ida
picking raspberries, which earned it a specific name *idaeus* in honour of the
mountain found near Troy in modern Turkey.

In his medicinal herbal *Botanologia Universalis Hibernica* (published 1735)
the Irish naturalist John K'Eogh recommended a variety of uses for
raspberry: '... an application of the flowers bruised in honey is beneficial for
the inflammation of the eyes, burning fever and boils, the fruit is good
for the heart and diseases of the mouth.'

The leaves of the plant continue to be used as eyewashes for conjunctivitis, mouthwashes for oral complaints and lotions for ulcers, wounds or
excessive vaginal discharge. The berries, which contain polyphenols, are
high in vitamins and have antioxidant and anti-inflammatory qualities used
by herbalists to reduce joint inflammation, cartilage damage, bone resorp-
tion and gastrointestinal disorders.

Oil made from raspberry seeds is rich in vitamin E, carotenes and
essential fatty acids, making it increasingly popular as a natural ingredient in
cosmetic skin products.

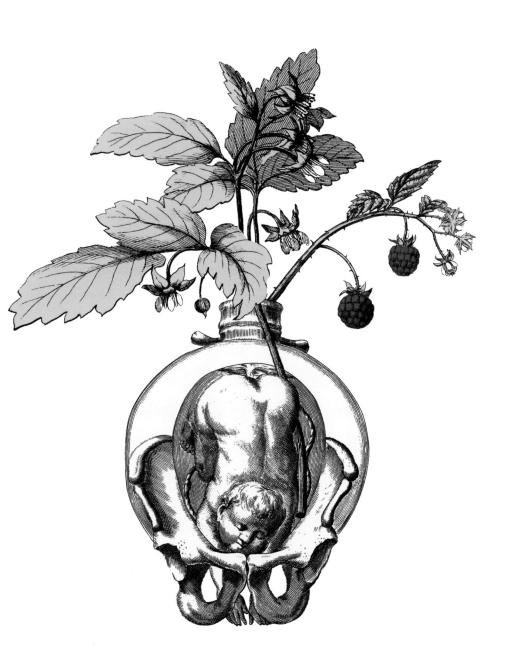

RASPBERRY LEAF • PELVIS

PENNYROYAL

Mentha pulegium

OTHER COMMON NAMES

royal thyme, pulegium, run-by-the-ground, lurk-in-the-ditch, pudding grass,
piliolerial, churchwort, flea mint, organ herb

Do not be fooled by the aromatic, mint-like charms of this perennial with its whorls of lilac flowers and creeping stems – generations of 'wise women' have drawn on its powers as a stimulant to induce abortions.

The Ancient Greek physician Dioscorides, whose five-volume encyclopaedia of herbal medicines was widely followed for fifteen centuries, claimed that pennyroyal provoked menstruation and labour. He wrote: 'Being boiled and drunk, it removes the menses, and expels the dead child and afterbirth...'.

Long since deemed far too toxic to be employed as a safe form of abortifacient, this native of Europe, Western Asia and North Africa is obviously to be avoided by pregnant women.

Despite its unsavoury reputation, various traditional healers have sought to derive positives from pennyroyal, by making distilled water from it to treat spasms, hysteria, nervous complaints, diarrhoea, flatulence and 'affections of the joints'. In 1597, John Gerard wrote that a 'garland of pennie royal made and worne about the head is of great force against the swimming of the head, and the pains and giddiness thereof'.

Like Gerard, modern herbalists sometimes prescribe pennyroyal as a treatment for headaches, although it is far more likely to be used in a similar way to peppermint: as a tonic to increase digestive secretions and reduce colic and flatulence. Pennyroyal tea tends to be employed as a throat wash or balm for general cold symptoms, while infusions might be proffered as treatments for itchiness and rheumatic conditions.

Pennyroyal's species name of *pulegium* is derived from the Latin word *pulex* ('flea'): its small, oval leaves were historically rubbed on dogs and cats as a flea repellent. The plant's leaves remain popular as a natural form of insect repellent as well as a make-shift treatment for horsefly, mosquito and wasp stings.

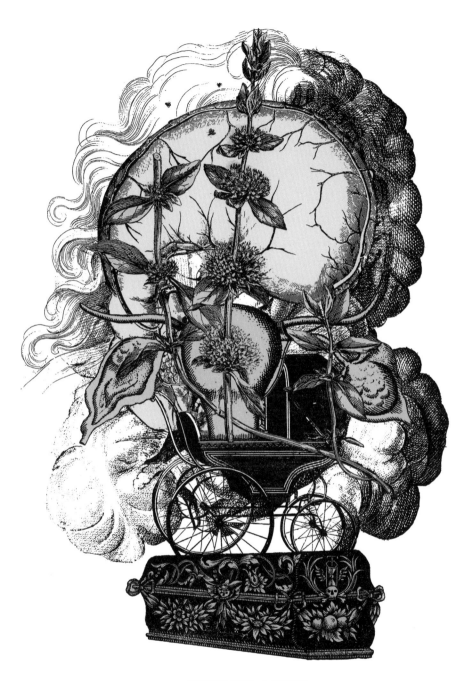

PENNYROYAL · PELVIS

GOLDENROD

Solidago virgaurea

OTHER COMMON NAMES
Aaron's rod, cast-the-spear, farewell summer

H ERBALISTS HAVE ALWAYS taken a flexible approach to the use of goldenrod, which is an antioxidant, diuretic and astringent. 'America's greatest inventor', Thomas Edison, successfully experimented with it in the 1920s in a bid to maximize the commercially valuable rubber content contained within its stems.

Native Americans chewed on the plant's toothed leaves to relieve sore throats or toothaches, and it has also been used to treat tuberculosis, diabetes, asthma, arthritis, chronic nasal catarrh and diarrhoea. The constant across the centuries has, however, remained its reputation as a healer of urinary complaints.

The seventeenth-century herbalist and physician Nicholas Culpeper once wrote of goldenrod: 'It is a sovereign wound-herb, inferior to none, both for inward and outward use. It is good to stay the immoderate flux of women's courses, the bloody flux, ruptures, ulcers in the mouth or throat, and in lotions to wash the privy parts in venereal cases.'

Modern herbalists use the plant to treat urinary tract infections, nephritis and cystitis, and it is regularly employed to help flush out kidney and bladder stones and to relieve backache brought on by renal conditions. The high levels of the organic chemical saponin in goldenrod act specifically against the *Candida* fungus, which is the cause of vaginal and oral thrush.

This hardy perennial likes waste ground and hillsides, and its branched spikes of golden yellow flowers (harvested in summer) are often responsible for the haze of colour seen growing by the sides of motorways. Edison would have approved of this ongoing link to the road network as he enjoyed driving a Model 'T' car gifted to him by his friend Henry Ford – one featuring tyres made from the 'goldenrod latex' that Edison himself had originally experimented with.

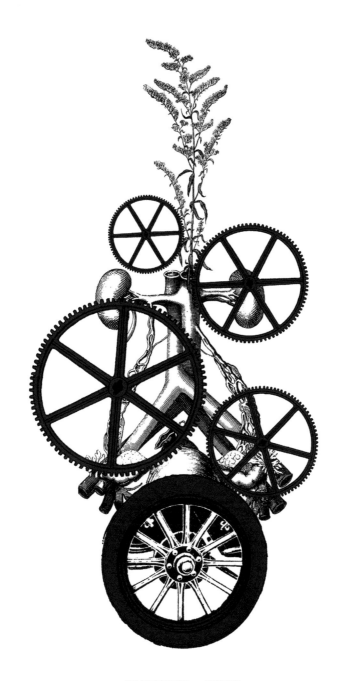

GOLDENROD · PELVIS

CHASTE TREE

Vitex agnus-castus

OTHER COMMON NAMES

monk's pepper, lygos, hemp tree, Abraham's tree,
chaste berry, tree of chastity

IN THE LATE fifth century BC, the Greek physician Hippocrates wrote: 'If blood flows from the womb, let the woman drink dark wine in which the leaves of the chaste tree have been steeped.' Approximately 2,400 years later (in the early part of the twentieth century), Hippocrates's reputation as an outstanding figure in the history of medicine would be underlined by a German doctor and scientist who had also become interested in this tree.

Gerhard Madaus was inspired by the work of the ancient healers and developed a new medicine from the dried berries of the large and aromatic shrub, which would be marketed as Agnolyt; it proved so successful that it has remained widely available ever since for the treatment of common female reproductive concerns.

Recent scientific research suggests that the berries of the chaste tree induce a subtle hormonal effect within the brain that leads to increased levels of dopamine and melatonin, improving regulation of the menstrual cycle and encouraging a better balance of hormones to address menopausal problems and raise fertility levels.

Popular in tablet or tincture form, the berries of this buddleja-like native of the Mediterranean can relieve spasms of menstrual pain and premenstrual syndrome and also reduce acne and migraines. They might be prescribed for polycystic ovary syndrome, fibroids and endometriosis, too.

As its most common name suggests, the chaste tree has long been associated with sacred rites of fertility and purity: Homer mentions it in *The Iliad* as a symbol of chastity, while Christian monks chewed on the leaves and ate the berries to reduce their libido. The plant's species name *agnus-castus* ('chaste lamb') may explain why the vestal virgins of Rome carried twigs from the tree around with them as a display of their purity.

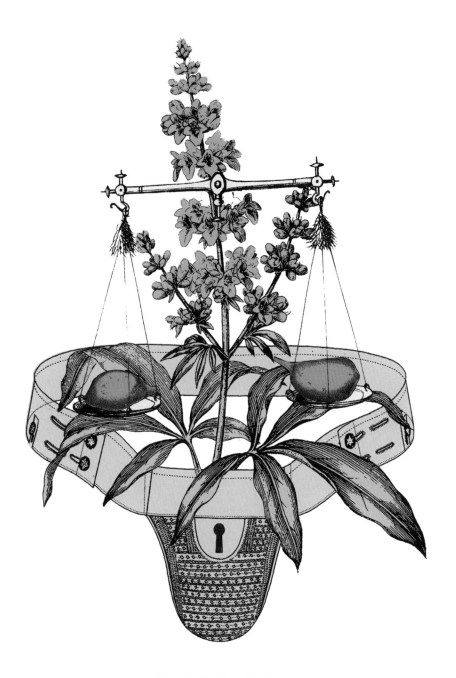

CHASTE TREE • PELVIS

CLEAVERS

Galium aparine

OTHER COMMON NAMES

aparine, grip grass, catchweed, cleaverwort, stick-a-back, sticky willy, stickyweed,
goose share, goose grass, goosebill, gosling weed, clivers, beggar lice, bedstraw,
robin-run-the-hedge, poor Robin, Robin-in-the-grass, coachweed, goode's hair,
hedge-burrs, clabber grass, milk sweet, sweethearts, scratchweed,
barweed, hedgeheriff, hariff, hayruff, hay reve

BEING CONSIDERED A valuable diuretic, cleavers is commonly drunk as a fresh juice to treat kidney stones, bladder stones and other urinary conditions such as cystitis – and if you live in a temperate part of the world it might be growing unappreciated as a weed in your garden or hedgerow right now.

This white-flowered annual has straggling, sticky, lightly hairy stems that climb unapologetically over other plants to reach their maximum potential of around 1.75m (6ft). Cleavers gets its name from the way it propagates, which involves clinging (or cleaving) on to animal fur or human clothing in a bid to disperse its seeds. Such common names as aparine, grip grass, cleaverwort and stickyweed reference the plant's habit of hooking and catching on to things.

Prescribed across the centuries as a diuretic and lymphatic tonic, the Ancient Greek physician Dioscorides considered it useful for countering weariness, and he described shepherds as making use of the hairy stems as sieves for straining milk.

Cleaver seeds have been found in Neolithic settlements, and it has been discovered that the plant was collected for livestock food while extracts were used to curdle milk into cheese – the genus name *Galium* being derived from the Greek word for 'milk'.

In addition to urinary treatments, the crushed plant parts are sometimes prescribed by herbalists as a poultice for sores and blisters. The leaves can be made into infused skin washes to treat conditions such as seborrhoea, eczema, psoriasis and sunburn, while tea-like tonics are used as hair rinses to help ease dandruff and also relieve insomnia or constipation.

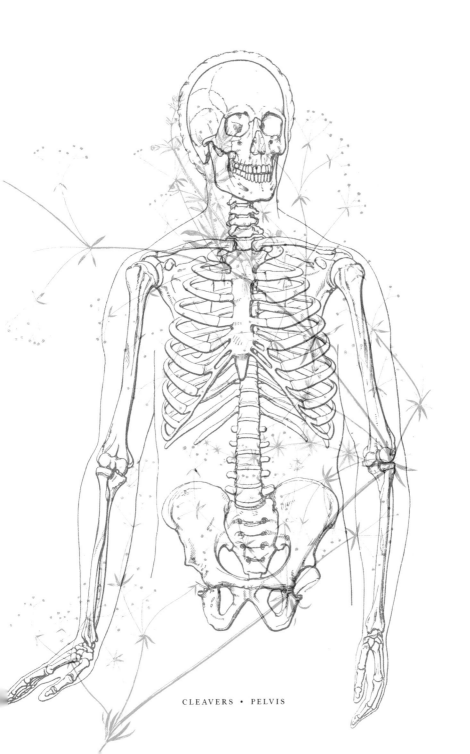

CLEAVERS · PELVIS

BARRENWORT

Epimedium grandiflorum

OTHER COMMON NAMES
horny goat weed, bishop's hat, fairy wings, *yin yang huo*

THE HIGHLY EVOCATIVE name of this short but hardy perennial is linked to its odd square and horn-like flower heads that appear in spring and belie the delicacy of the wing-like leaves that provide its traditional source of power.

The Chinese name for the plant is *yin yang huo* ('licentious goat plant'), and it has been picked and used for centuries in China as a cure for male impotence and low libido.

It is claimed that two chemical compounds contained within barrenwort (icariin and phytoestrogens) act as a support for both men and women of a certain age: icariin is reputed to be responsible for increasing blood flow to improve male sexual function; and phytoestrogens acts like the female hormone oestrogen to help post-menopausal women with a variety of complaints from low sex drive to joint and bone problems.

Studies have shown that barrenwort raises adrenaline, noradrenaline, serotonin and dopamine levels in animals, with the increased levels of dopamine most likely to be responsible for setting off any chain reaction that could lead to a release of the male sex hormone testosterone. Further modern research has suggested that the herb may increase sensitivity in nerve endings, which could explain its popularity as an aphrodisiac, but all of this research is limited.

On a less provocative note, barrenwort is known to dilate blood vessels and have potential as a treatment for coronary heart disease, asthma, bronchitis, sinusitis and kidney problems including frequent urination.

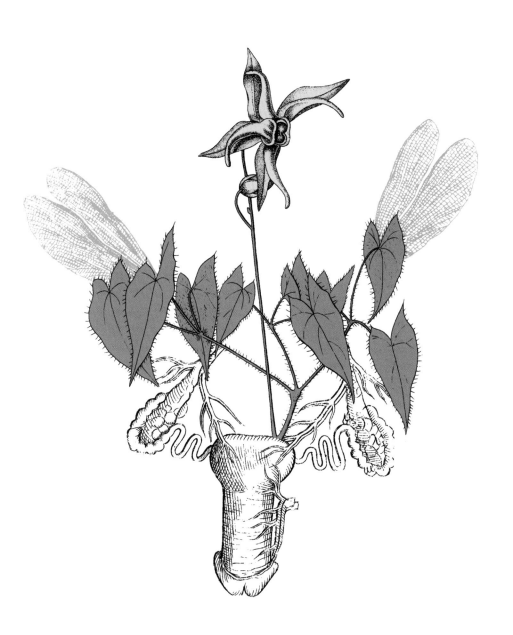

BARRENWORT • PELVIS

JUNIPER

Juniperus communis

OTHER COMMON NAMES
juniper bush, bastard killer, common juniper,
gin berry, geneva, gin plant

THIS SMALL AND slow-growing evergreen develops aromatic, spiky leaves, while its deep blue berries of juniper grow only on female plants and are traditionally associated with reproduction.

Native Americans used juniper berries as a female contraceptive, and the Ancient Greek physician Dioscorides recommended (in his herbal *De Materia Medica* of AD 50–70) that the berries be 'crushed and put on the penis or vagina before intercourse, as a contraceptive'.

Known to stimulate menstruation and increase related bleeding, this plant was once used in parts of rural England as an inducer of abortions and given the unofficial title of bastard killer. It should clearly be avoided by pregnant women.

Now prescribed as a diuretic with strong antiseptic properties, it is also seen as valuable for treating cystitis, helping fluid retention and for supporting those suffering with chronic arthritis.

Native across the northern hemisphere, it grows widely on moorlands, mountain slopes and in coniferous forests.

Renowned as a flavouring in the making of gin, juniper berries are also consumed in meat dishes and marinades. In a practice dating back to the Ancient Greeks, oil made from extracts of the plant is still used to massage aching muscles of athletes and increase their stamina.

There are sixty species of juniper, although only one variety appears to have been used medicinally: *J. communis*. We can shed no light on whether such specifics of species were important to those who traditionally threw a sprig of juniper on to the fire to ward off evil spirits.

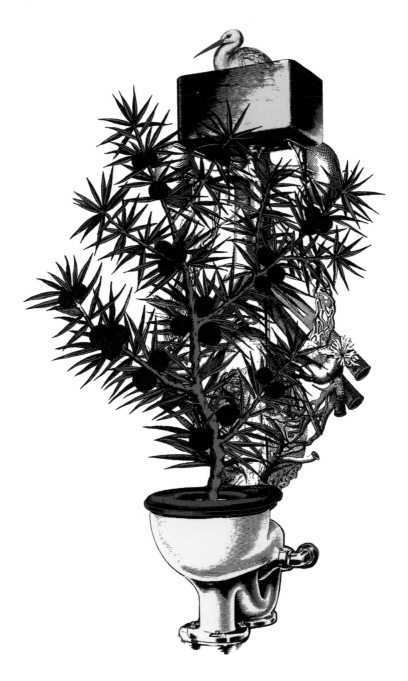

JUNIPER • PELVIS

CRAMPBARK

Viburnum opulus

OTHER COMMON NAMES
kalyna, guelder rose, highbush cranberry, snowball tree, snowball bush,
water elder, dog eller, dog rowan, European cranberry bush, gatten, gatten tree,
marsh alder, ople tree, red elder, rose elder, whitten tree

A S I T S N A M E suggests, this tall flowering shrub is mainly used to relieve cramps – and especially painful menstruation caused by the over-contraction of muscles. It has remained highly valued by American Indians for its ability to ease general muscle pains across the body.

It is not just in America that the shrub has had a significant impact – the Slavic nations are particularly attached to crampbark, or *kalyna* as it is known across Eastern Europe. A national symbol of Russia, it also features repeatedly in Ukrainian folklore and the pagan mythology of the wider region – including playing a leading role in the story of the birth of the Universe and 'Fire Trinity' (the sun, moon and stars).

Although there has been little clinical research undertaken into the medical value of crampbark, it remains popular with herbalists and has been recognized since 1960 by the United States Pharmacopeia and National Formulary (USP–NF) as a successful remedy for nervous conditions and asthma.

Native to Europe and parts of Asia, the shrub grows in woodland, hedges and thickets and enjoys damp soil. Gardeners see it as a seasonal 'beacon' as its white flowers bloom in spring and its bright clusters of berries arrive in autumn.

The berries of crampbark are said by Eastern Europeans to represent blood lines and the enduring strength of family ties and are highly valued by the various species of birds that love to feast on them.

Herbalists tend to favour external application of crampbark for muscle treatments, and internal ingestion for most of the other maladies with which it is associated, such as arthritis, blood circulation, relief from intestinal and uterus pain, colic, respiratory problems and (more recently) kidney stones.

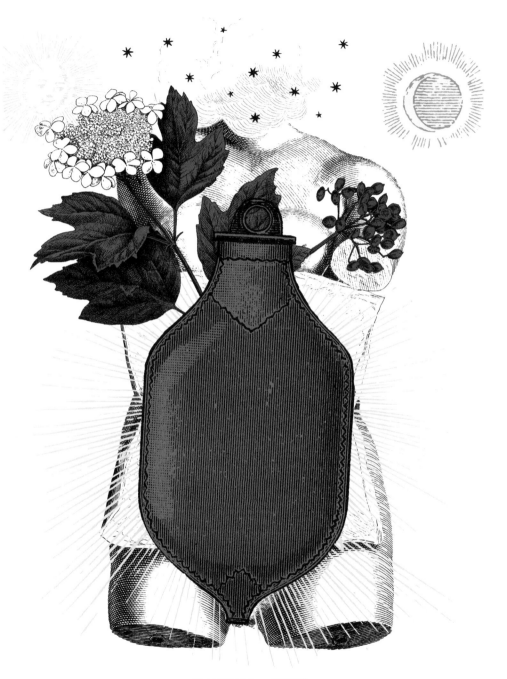

CRAMPBARK • PELVIS

RED CLOVER

Trifolium pratense

OTHER COMMON NAMES
meadow trefoil, bee bread, cow grass, purple clover, three-leafed grass,
purple wort, sugar plums, common clover,
marl grass, pinkies, suckles

WIDELY CULTIVATED BY farmers as a fodder crop to make hay and improve soil, the flower heads of red clover are also thought to be of direct value to a range of human conditions linked to low oestrogen levels.

This perennial, which is loved by bees, has hairy, upright stems, oval leaves and purple, egg-shaped flowers. Native to Europe and Asia, it was historically used as a treatment for breast cancer: a strong and concentrated decoction would be applied to the site of a tumour to encourage it to 'grow outwards' and leave the body. Unfortunately, modern research into the prevention and treatment of breast cancer has not suggested there is any value to such traditional uses.

Being high in phytoestrogen compounds, including isoflavones, which can help regulate and boost falling oestrogen and other hormone levels in both women and men, red clover is most commonly associated with the treatment of menopausal symptoms in females, such as hot flushes.

Extracts of this plant are thought to have a protective impact on the human heart and circulation, while also countering bone loss and preventing osteoporosis. Less dramatically, it is employed as an expectorant, cough treatment and aid for skin conditions.

Clovers were seen as sacred by ancient northern peoples such as the Celts, who believed they represented the ongoing evolution and rebirth of life in all its natural forms. The herb continues to be seen as a bringer of luck, although few have quite the same levels of expectation as their forebears – especially when it comes to the need for protection from witches and impish fairies.

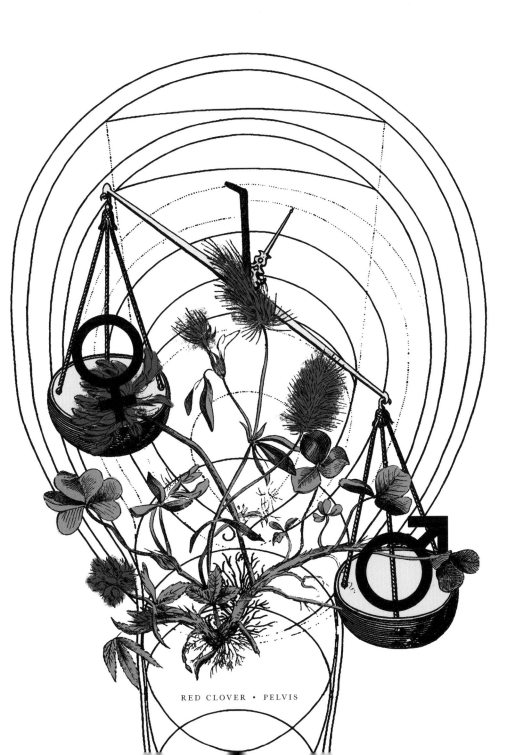

RED CLOVER • PELVIS

CRANBERRY

Vaccinium macrocarpon

OTHER COMMON NAMES

American cranberry, large cranberry, wonder berry, crane berry

FOR NATIVE AMERICANS such as the Iroquois, Algonquin, Ojibwa and Chippewa this small, slender evergreen was a common traditional source of nutrition and a medical cleanser, and they called it 'crane berry' because of the large birds that regularly came to feed on it.

Now recognized as a classic remedy for urinary tract infections, the berries of this shrub are just as likely to be recommended by doctors working in general medical practice as herbalists. The red, oval berries have antibiotic properties and, scientific studies show, are rich in antioxidants as well as vitamin C.

Among cranberry's most popular medicinal uses are the treatment of poor urinary flow; prevention of urinary stones; cure of enlarged prostates, bladder and kidney infections, cystitis and urethritis; and the cleansing of infected urinary tubes.

Despite the undisputable health benefits of this shrub, it remains best known internationally as a sauce to accompany cooked fowl at seasonal feasts – a tradition tied to American folklore and the first 'Thanksgiving', at which it is claimed the early pilgrims would have used crushed cranberries to sweeten their festive fayre. The colonists had been taught how to sweeten cranberries by Native Americans, who had been using the same berries for food, dye and medicine long before they ever broke bread with the pilgrims.

One of only three commercially grown fruits native to the USA, cranberry thrives in acid soil and wet boggy ground. The traditional Swedish habit of drinking the unsweetened berries as a tart and acidic refresher has now caught on in many parts of the world, resulting in it being cultivated widely where conditions are suitable.

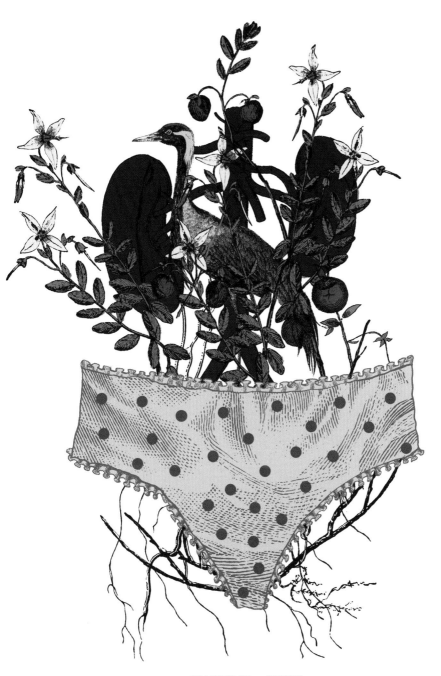

CRANBERRY · PELVIS

VERVAIN

Verbena officinalis

OTHER COMMON NAMES

common vervain, common verbena, *ma bian cao*, herb of grace, herb of the Cross,
holy herb, holy wort, *herba sacra*, enchanter's plant, herb of enchantment,
Juno's tears, pigeon's grass, divine wood, mosquito plant,
wizard's herb, iron herb

VERVAIN WAS REGARDED as a sacred herb in many early cultures.
The Ancient Egyptians believed that it originated from the tears
of Isis, the goddess of fertility, while the Ancient Greeks, Romans
and druids used it during sacrificial ceremonies.

Superstitions abound about this slender perennial, including a Christian
belief that a blessing must be given before it is picked because it was used to
stem the flow of Christ's blood at the crucifixion. Many of its common
names, such as holy herb and herb of the Cross, reference this belief.

In the Middle Ages vervain was carried for good luck and would go on to
appear in love potions and aphrodisiacs as well as in ointments, to disperse
demons. Metalsmiths once used the plant during procedures to harden
steel, and in some European countries (such as Holland, Germany,
Denmark, and Slovakia) it is still known as iron herb.

Culpeper said of vervain: 'This is a herb of Venus, and excellent for the
womb to strengthen and remedy all the cold griefs of it.' His opinion holds
good for many, and particularly in Chinese medicine where it is sometimes
prescribed for premenstrual tension and other conditions relating to the
menstrual cycle – in addition to promoting contractions of the womb's
muscles and boosting of breast milk production.

Featuring stiff stems with spikes of white flowers, vervain grows wild
across Europe, North America, North and East Africa, China, Japan and
Australia, and is harvested just prior to flowering in summer. The aerial
elements are used for medicinal purposes, which might include migraines,
nervous tension, anxiety, mild depression, absorption, jaundice, asthma, flu
and insomnia.

Although a plant of clear value, it should be noted that the levels of the
bitter-tasting chemical compound verbenalin contained within it may cause
vomiting if consumed in high doses.

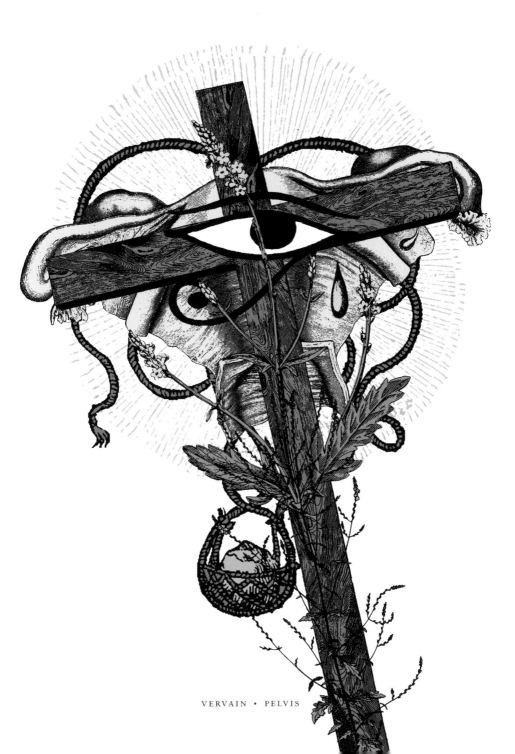

VERVAIN · PELVIS

CORN SILK

Zea mays

OTHER COMMON NAMES
mother's hair, Indian corn, maize jagnog, Turkish corn,
yu mi xu, stigmata maydis, sweetcorn

THIS PLANT IS valued as a treatment for a wide array of conditions. The Aztecs drank corn silk tea to combat dysentery and increase breast milk production, but it is most likely to be used by modern herbalists as a treatment for urinary conditions.

Being a demulcent and diuretic, corn silk can help those suffering from acute cystitis, prostate disorders and bladder irritations. It can be consumed fresh but is often dried before being taken as a pill or tea: the dried extracts can be added to hot water and drunk up to five times a day.

Originally a native crop of the Andes and Americas, corn silk has been cultivated in Central and South America for more than 4,000 years as a source of cheap food – and cherished for just as long by followers of traditional Native American, Mayan, Incan and Chinese medicine.

Now rebranded as sweetcorn and grown across the globe, the fine, thread-like fronds that are wrapped around the cobs of this annual grass are what are referred to as corn silk. Reaching up to 3m (10ft) in height, the plume-like flowers are male, but it is the less visually impressive female flowers that produce the more useful cobs.

Chinese physicians still prescribe corn silk in a drink to treat fluid retention and jaundice, and it is used in some cultures to treat heart disease, malaria, kidney stones, swellings, sores and boils. Known to contain high levels of carotenoids, which are thought to protect the eye from oxidative damage and age-related macular degeneration, it is clear that adherents of this humble healer may enjoy benefits that far outweigh their expectations.

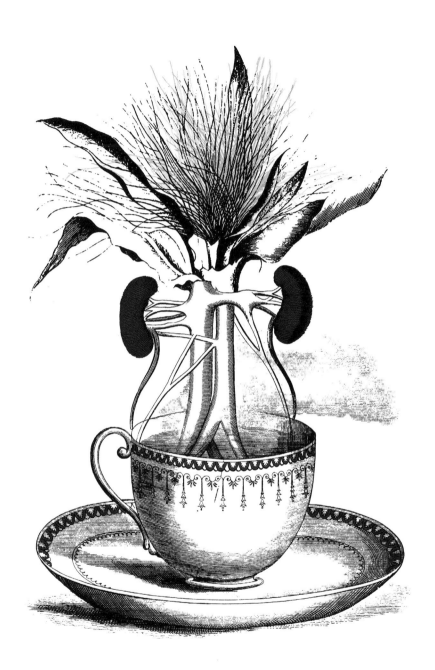

CORN SILK • PELVIS

FENUGREEK

Trigonella foenum-graecum

OTHER COMMON NAMES
methi, shanbalileh, Greek clover, Greek hay

THE ANCIENT EGYPTIAN medicinal texts known as the *Ebers Papyrus* (1,550 BC) records the seeds of fenugreek as working to induce childbirth. It has continued to be prescribed for all manner of gynaecological and birthing problems ever since and is thus a staple of medicine cabinets in most parts of the world.

This strongly aromatic annual with pea-like flowers and sickle-shaped pods will happily grow on wasteland. Native to Asia, it is now widely cultivated commercially – particularly in India and Africa where it is seen as something of a 'cure-all' herb.

The fresh, trifoliate leaves of fenugreek are often consumed in curries and teas, but it is the seeds (which are harvested in autumn) that are most prized for their medicinal value. Commonly used to treat cramping period pains, polycystic ovary syndrome, infections of the uterus and inflammation of the vagina, the seeds are also prescribed as a way of encouraging a reluctant baby into the world and as a booster for breast milk.

High in vitamins, this versatile plant is claimed to be as good as quinine at lowering a temperature brought on by fever, while also having the power to soothe gastritis and gastric ulcers, lower cholesterol, encourage weight gain among convalescing patients and anorexics, and control insulin resistance and late-onset diabetes.

The Latin name for fenugreek is translated as 'Greek hay', which is in reference to its use as a fortifier of cattle feed. The bovines do not know how lucky they are.

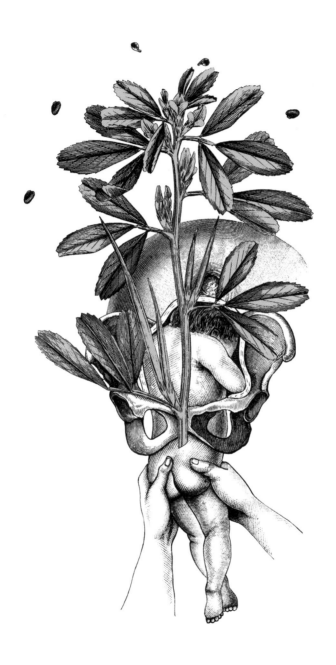

FENUGREEK • PELVIS

CHINESE PEONY

Paeonia lactiflora

OTHER COMMON NAMES
peony, common garden peony,
shao yao, bai shao yao

CULTIVATED THROUGHOUT north-east China and Inner Mongolia, this upright perennial is one of the herbs sometimes featured in a popular 'Four Herbs Soup' – a Chinese tonic for women that is taken as a cure for a range of gynaecological problems from cramps to dizziness.

Specifically the roots of peony contain phytoestrogen compounds and hormone-balancing chemicals that may well help with menstrual disorders such as heavy or irregular periods and bleeding, period pains and cramps, and poor fertility. Sometimes prescribed with liquorice (see page 92), it has been shown to support regular ovulation and lower the kind of raised testosterone levels that are typically found among sufferers of polycystic ovary syndrome.

Containing antispasmodic and anti-inflammatory properties, peony root has performed well in some clinical trials as an aid for rheumatoid arthritis. The constituent thought to be most responsible for the success – paeoniflorin – is also considered helpful for lowering blood pressure, increasing blood flow to the heart and reducing the risk of clotting.

Popular claims that this plant can boost mental functions such as spatial awareness are not backed up by research, although a recent study did conclude that paeoniflorin has a beneficial effect on the gut, which can in turn have a positive chemical effect on anxiety and depression.

The roots of white peony are harvested after four or five years and tend to appear commercially as capsules, powders or tinctures. Picked during the Middle Ages as a protection against 'the evil eye', in American folk magic the plant was used to hold misfortune at bay or to break a jinx.

It is considered a symbol of prosperity in modern Japan, where traditionally women who partake of peony root on a regular basis are said to become as radiant as its blooms.

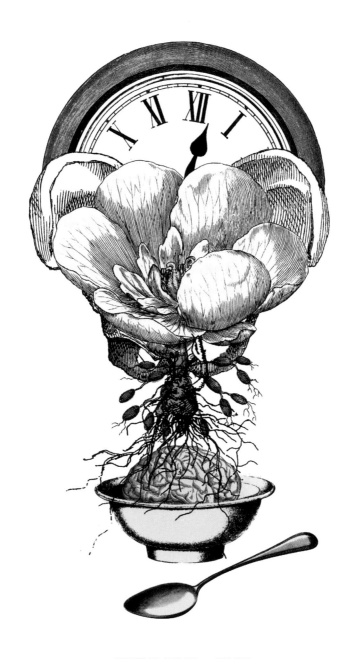

CHINESE PEONY • PELVIS

BLACK COHOSH

Actaea racemosa, syn. *Cimicifuga racemosa*

squaw root, slack bugbane, black snakeroot, baneberry, fairy candle,
deerweed, feather wands, rattle root, rattleweed, rattlesnake weed,
summer rockets, swan's neck, Virginia snakeroot

NATIVE AMERICAN HEALERS have used extracts of this herbaceous perennial for centuries as a balm for menstrual and menopausal problems. Modern studies have provided scientific provenance for their actions – many of the issues associated with such complaints are linked to low oestrogen levels, and while black cohosh does not contain oestrogen it is said to stimulate an action in the brain that boosts levels of the chemical within the body.

This plant stands tall, reaching up to 2.5m (8ft) in height, and prefers shady spots in woods and hedgerows in North America. Herbalists use its roots more than its lance-like, musty smelling leaves or tall and creamy flower spears.

European settlers in America and Canada learnt from Native North Americans, and the plant went on to appear in the *United States Pharmacopeia* (USP) under the name of black snakeroot. It has subsequently been used to treat snakebites, inflamed lungs and pain from childbirth – as well as rheumatic problems and high blood pressure.

Some modern studies have suggested that extracts of black cohosh might help slow the development of osteoporosis and breast cancer and have future potential in the treatment of polycystic ovary syndrome, but this research is far from conclusive and remains contentious – there have been alternative studies suggesting the plant may speed up breast cancer and cause liver damage.

It may be wise to take the disagreeable odour and bitter taste of black cohosh as a warning to resist drawing on its obvious powers without first taking advice from a professional physician.

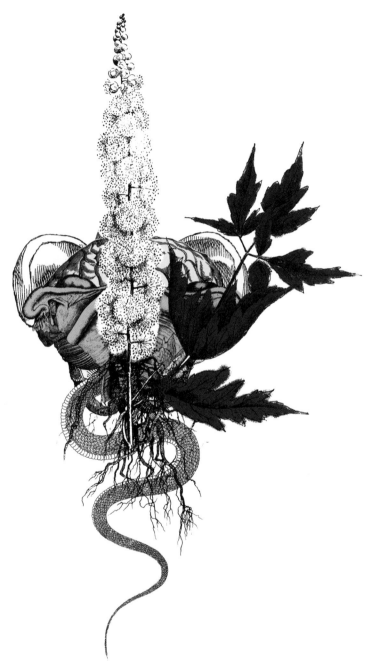

BLACK COHOSH • PELVIS

SKELETON

bones, muscles, skin

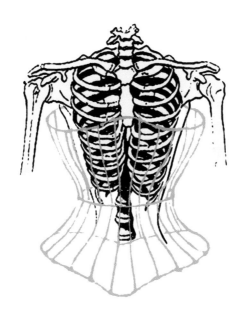

YARROW

Achillea millefolium

nosebleed, woundwort, thousand leaf, carpenter's weed, noble yarrow,
common yarrow, devil's nettle, hundred-leaved grass, lace plant,
milfoil, nose pepper, old man's pepper, sanguinary,
savory tea, soldier's woundwort

Being a plant worthy of warriors, yarrow was commonly carried into battle by Ancient Greek and Roman soldiers, while Achilles used it to staunch the bleeding of his men's wounds (earning it the name of *Achillea*).

Laboratory studies indicate that yarrow may help dilate blood vessels and arrest bleeding in much the same way that conventional angiotensin-converting enzyme (ACE) inhibitors do when prescribed for high blood pressure. The plant is also used by herbalists to regulate menstrual cycles and associated bleeding, as well as a wide array of other treatments including colds, flu, digestion, colic, hay fever, varicose veins and fevers.

As well as being a friend to the war-like, yarrow is also referred to as carpenter's weed for similar reasons – tradesmen, like woodworkers, used it to stem bleeds from their work-related cuts.

In folklore, this native from the northern hemisphere was said to prevent (but not cure) baldness. Druids used it to divine the weather while young girls used it to foresee the perfect love match – believing that if they tickled their nose with a spray of the small white flowers and got a nosebleed their chosen one would prove true. They might also place a leaf under their pillow if they needed help in their search for love.

Yarrow is known as a 'plant doctor' for good reason: if planted near unhealthier counterparts, secretions from its roots help trigger an immune response among its ailing neighbours. For similar reasons it makes a great accelerant in composts, fertilizers and fungicides. It is not always so popular with gardeners as it often takes root in a lawn or in the cracks of paths.

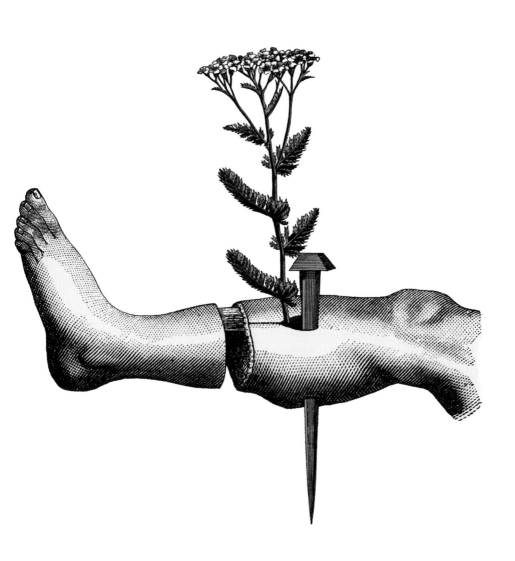

YARROW · SKELETON

CHICKWEED

Stellaria media

OTHER COMMON NAMES
starweed, star chickweed, adder's mouth chickweed, Indian chickweed,
satin flower, scarped, starwort, stitchwort, tongue grass, white bird's-eye,
little star lady, bird herb, chick whittle, chicken's meat, chickenwort,
cluckweed, craches, maruns, winterweed

THIS COMMON SOURCE of cheap feed for fowl is also capable of relieving many a human scratch, rash, insect bite or general skin irritation. From burns to boils and abscesses to eczema, slender-stemmed chickweed boasts an impressive medical portfolio.

Characterized by its small, star-like, white flowers, chickweed is an annual that can be found in most parts of the world. Being something of a sun worshipper, it likes to 'sleep' during the night and on cloudy days and will tend to fully unfold its leaves only when the sun comes out.

Herbalists often present chickweed in the form of a soothing poultice or ointment, and the famous twelfth-century German abbess, herbalist, mystic and musician Saint Hildegard of Bingen (who drew heavily on Eastern practices) recommended that it be applied directly as a treatment for wounds and sores. One of its more common names, stitchwort, also implies that it was incorporated into the process of stitching wounds.

Chickweed's healing powers are probably due to its high saponin content, which is thought to give it a high level of interaction with the components of cell membranes. As well as being administered externally, it is sometimes presented as a juice – chickweed water having long been imbibed (most likely due to its laxative qualities) as a remedy for obesity.

Fresh chickweed can be eaten in salads to help address an iron deficiency, but it is far more likely to appear as part of the diet of your pet as it helps sooth digestive tracts and encourages the expulsion of hairballs.

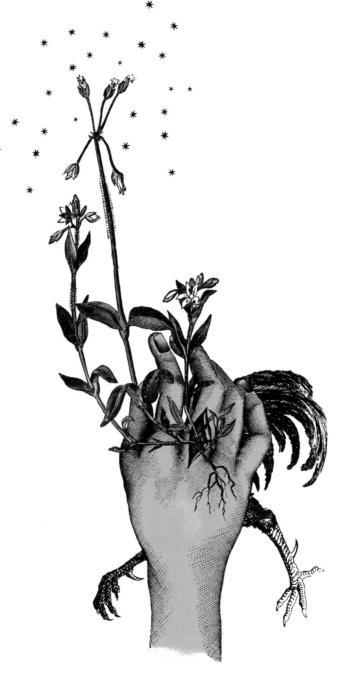

CHICKWEED • SKELETON

COMFREY

Symphytum officinale

OTHER COMMON NAMES

knitbone, boneset, slippery root, blackwort, bruisewort, consound, healing herb,
gum plant, knit back, ass ear, miracle herb, wallwort, knotherb, churchbells,
Abraham-Isaac-and-Jacob, Saracen's root

THE HEALING POWERS of this perennial are linked to the high
levels of allantoin that it contains – a compound usually
extracted from the plant's roots or leaves that has been shown to help
stimulate and repair damaged cell tissue.

Believed to have been brought to mainland Europe by Crusaders, who had
discovered that its secretions worked as a form of plaster for setting bones,
comfrey's name may well be derived from the Latin *confero* ('knitting
together') – all of which tallies rather nicely with other common names for
the plant such as knitbone, boneset and knit back.

The Ancient Greek physician Dioscorides prescribed comfrey as a healer
of wounds and broken bones while Elizabethan physicians were never
without a herb once seen as the panacea for all ills. Modern herbalists draw
on the plant to relieve pain and inflammation caused by injury and
degenerative symptoms related to rheumatoid arthritis and osteoarthritis. In
Germany it is still in common use for sprains, bruises and sports injuries,
and recent studies indicate that its value in tissue repair, as well as an
anti-inflammatory for sprains, osteoarthritis and lower back pain, are not
without foundation.

This plant will live happily in most conditions and can be used to treat
insect bites, burns, scars, skin inflammation, acne and mastitis. It has thick,
foxglove-like leaves and its unfurling pink or purple bell flowers are a
favourite of bees and much-loved by gardeners and allotment owners, who
often create compost accelerants and plant feed by steeping the leaves over
long periods.

Usually proffered as an external cream or oil, comfrey should never be
consumed because elements of the plant, especially its roots, can be highly
toxic for the liver and, according to some modern research, potentially
carcinogenic.

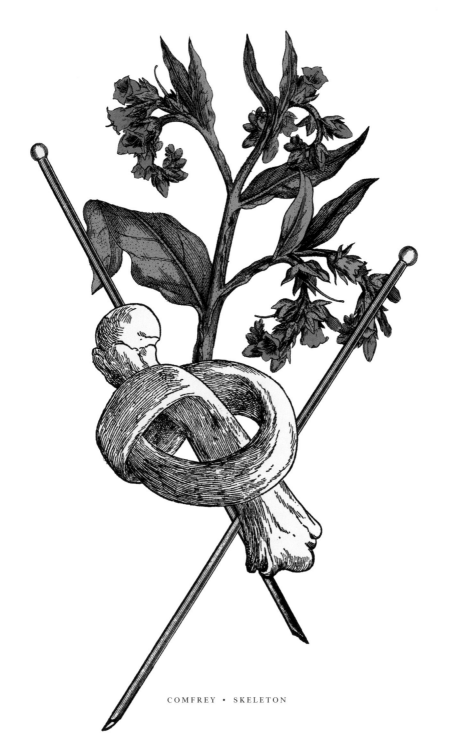

COMFREY • SKELETON

ALOE VERA

Aloe vera

OTHER COMMON NAMES
bitter aloes, medicine plant, burn plant, Cape aloes,
sea houseleek, Curaçao aloé, Barbados aloe

THE BACKSTORIES OF the humblest of herbs can often provide cause to pause, and a modern house plant cherished for centuries across different continents is not about to buck the trend.

Cultivated and growing wild around the equator, the regenerative powers of aloe vera have been as valued by the embalmers of the Egyptian pharaohs as the Ancient Roman physicians who treated the wounds of the gladiators. Cleopatra is said to have incorporated extracts of aloe vera into her beauty regime, while the Ancient Greeks revered the plant as a harbinger of good fortune and health.

Commonly applied externally in skin ointments for wounds, burns, sores, eczema, psoriasis and more, it is the gel found within aloe vera's fleshy and sword-like leaves that is key – containing antibacterial properties that provide a protective barrier around damaged skin, promoting the healing process and offering a soothing balm.

As a clear example of this evergreen's healing power, if you pick a leaf and leave it in the sun for weeks it will return to its fresh plump state when immersed in water.

Often consumed as a juice for digestive and kidney disorders, clinical studies have shown that aloe vera can also help with mouth ulcers and bronchial asthmas – and there is ongoing research into whether it could have a positive role to play in the treatment of human immunodeficiency virus (HIV), diabetes and cancers.

The plant can grow to around 60cm (2ft) in height and, while popular with the world's domestic gardeners, it is usually harvested commercially in hotter climes because the potency of its main healing ingredient, anthraquinone, is increased by the warmth of the sun's rays.

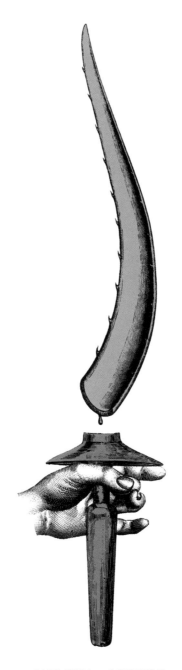

ALOE VERA • SKELETON

WILD CELERY

Apium graveolens

OTHER COMMON NAMES

smaller eggs, smallage, ach, ache, celery, celery seed, marche,
marsh parsley, smalledge, sweet parsley, Venus's herb

ONE OF THE oldest vegetables in recorded history is wild celery, which was collected as a food by the Ancient Egyptians and its remains found in Tutankhamun's tomb. The cultivar of celery that most people now consume was introduced in the seventeenth century by Italian farmers.

Being known for its cleansing properties and ability to help dispose of uric acid, urates and other wastes that can cause pain and inflammation in gout and rheumatic conditions, wild celery seeds are often prescribed in infusions to treat such complaints. The seeds can also help to improve blood circulation to ease muscle and joint pain, which might explain why the Ancient Greeks valued this vegetable so highly – honouring their champion athletes with crowns made from its leaves. On a more sombre note, the Greek writer Plutarch mentions it was used to decorate graves, and the dead were often crowned with it, a double symbolism of death and victory.

Native to many European countries, wild celery grows in marshlands and has small hollow stalks that bloom with flat and umbrella-like masses of tiny white flowers. Its botanical name is derived from the Latin *apis* ('bee') and *graveolens* ('heavily scented'). As might be expected, the plant is something of a favourite with bees.

Wild celery contains the compound luteolin, which can reduce inflammation in the brain and benefit cognitive health, and modern studies have shown this engenders a calming effect on the central nervous system and is a promoter of restful sleep. The plant is often prescribed as a blood-thinning tea to lower cholesterol levels, while its antiseptic and diuretic qualities also make it effective in the treatment of urinary conditions.

In India, wild celery is used to treat hiccups and flatulence, which bodes well for the soups and stews it is incorporated into in France – where the more concentrated flavour of wild celery is favoured over modern cultivars.

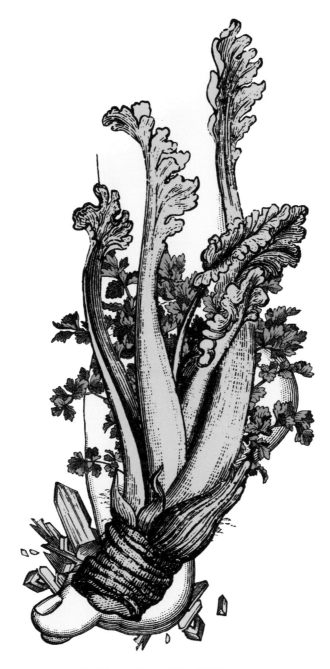

WILD CELERY • SKELETON

BROADLEAF PLANTAIN

Plantago major

OTHER COMMON NAMES
greater plantain, rat tail plantain, waybread, waybroad,
white man's foot, Englishman's foot

K NOWN IN GAELIC as 'the healing plant' because of its power to treat wounds and bruises, this treasured perennial is included in the Anglo-Saxon *Lacnunga* – a tenth-century medical treatise that lists the key herbs for treating infections and poisons.

Given its reputation, broadleaf plantain was an obvious choice for the medical bags of physicians accompanying expeditions to explore and colonize new territories – with Native Americans even naming the plant Englishman's foot or 'white man's foot' because of the way it seemed to spring up by pathways wherever the early English settlers established themselves. Further exploration of their own would see Native Americans go on to use it as a remedy for rattlesnake bites.

Native to Europe and temperate Asia, where it is often found by roadsides and on meadowland, the plant's rosettes of lush green leaves are gathered in summer and best used fresh for anti-inflammatory properties that help staunch blood flow and repair damaged skin tissue. Broadleaf plantain roots can also be mashed and put on bee stings, skin irritations, ulcers, burns and minor bleeding cuts.

Commonly presented in ointments or lotions, including the treatment of haemorrhoids, fistulae and ulcers, modern herbalists may also prescribe broadleaf plantain products for internal digestion to treat conditions such as gastritis, peptic ulcers, diarrhoea, dysentery, irritable bowel syndrome, respiratory catarrh, loss of voice and urinary tract bleeding.

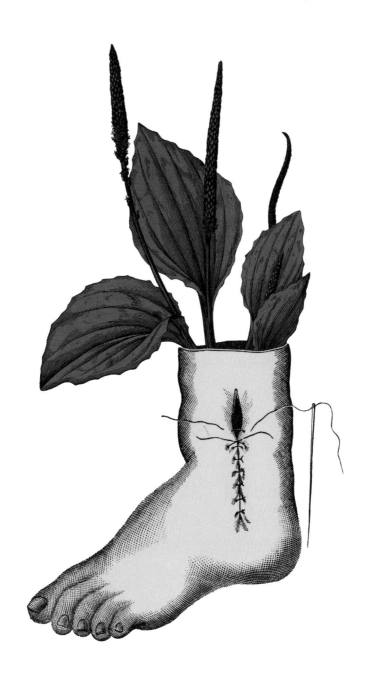

BROADLEAF PLANTAIN • SKELETON

CABBAGE

Brassica oleracea

OTHER COMMON NAMES

coleworts, wild cabbage, collards, field cabbage

BEING A POPULAR natural remedy for skin inflammation and swelling, the humble cabbage has been a go-to for generations of breast-feeding mums troubled by mastitis and engorgement.

And in this case, the old wives' tale is supported by modern research – keeping a chilled cabbage leaf in your bra for 20 minutes does appear to deliver a similar amount of pain relief as a hot compress.

Another traditional form of poultice is to cut off the midrib of a cooked leaf, iron it and place it (while still hot) on the area of skin that is the source of your ailment. This process is said to be good for blisters, although the fresh (uncooked) leaves of the plant are also used for suppuration purposes in some treatments.

Such practices have been utilized by generations of healers and are tied to the high levels of glutamine and amino acid harboured within the leaf – both of which have an anti-inflammatory effect when applied directly to sensitive skin tissue.

Cabbage is seen by modern herbalists as a good source of vitamins A and C (as well as iron, calcium and phosphorus). Despite its reputation for 'windiness' when eaten raw or drunk as a fresh juice, cabbage cleanses the digestive tract and is popular as a salve for stomach diseases, obesity, gastric and duodenal ulcers, haemorrhoids and the elimination of worms.

Other common uses for cabbage include poultices for facial neuralgia, rheumatic pains and aphonia (voice loss due to disease of the larynx) and for breaking down toxins in the liver – tallying with the Ancient Roman belief that cabbage could deliver a good hangover cure.

Factor in the main value of this compact biennial as a cheap source of nutrition, and there is more than enough evidence to show that the historic habit of using the name of cabbage in vain (as slang for a fool or stupid person or someone in an exhausted or vegetative state) has been nothing less than a gross miscarriage of botanical justice.

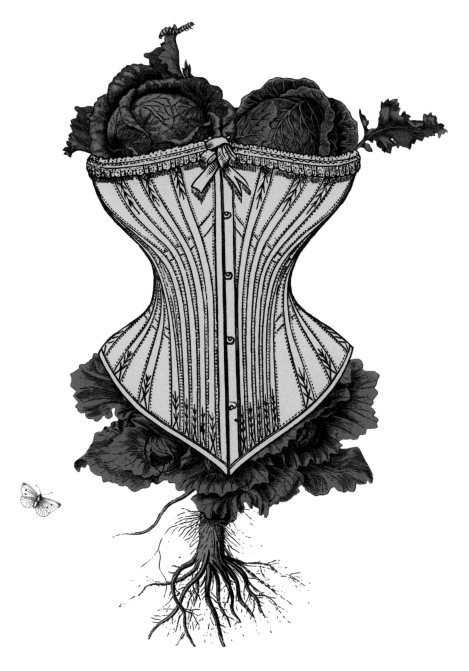

CABBAGE · SKELETON

NETTLE

Urtica dioica

OTHER COMMON NAMES
common nettle, stinging nettle, burn nettle, burn weed, burn hazel,
devil's leaf, devil's plaything, stinger, great nettle

ALTHOUGH COMMONLY associated with creating discomfort courtesy of its acidic 'sting', medicinal herbalists know that there are far more positives than negatives to this seemingly omnipotent plant.

With a creeping root system that enables it to spread with impunity, nettle is found all over the world. The stems have been used for fabric making for thousands of years, with the remains of bodies unearthed in a Bronze Age grave in Denmark (excavated in the nineteenth century) wrapped in nettle cloth. The Ancient Romans brought a species of nettle with them on their expeditions into northern Europe, which they apparently used to flog their arms and legs in a bid to keep their circulation going during the cold months. The plant remains a key tonic for the winter months thanks to high levels of the mineral boron, which is deemed helpful for easing rheumatic and arthritic conditions.

A diuretic, nettle is also seen as providing a good level of support for anaemia, although studies into its effects on osteoporosis have provided mixed results. Clinical trials have, however, shown that the plant's roots can reduce prostate enlargement and ease lower urinary tract symptoms.

Also containing antihistamine and anti-inflammatory compounds, extracts of the plant are used to treat hay fever and to alleviate bronchial and nasal obstructions, as well as an astringent to stop nosebleeds, heavy menstrual bleeds and reduce blood loss from wounds.

Spinach-like in flavour, nettle is often foraged for juices, soups and teas. Those who take on the challenge are reminded to wear gloves and to make sure that a supply of dock leaves, sorrel, rosemary, mint or sage is at hand as a balm for the inevitable 'burn' delivered when the tiny hairs of its leaves are disturbed.

When left steeped in water for several weeks, nettles make a very nutritious plant fertilizer. Claims that it can also feed hair follicles to prevent hair loss are about as reputable as the traditional belief that the plant provides a dwelling place for elves.

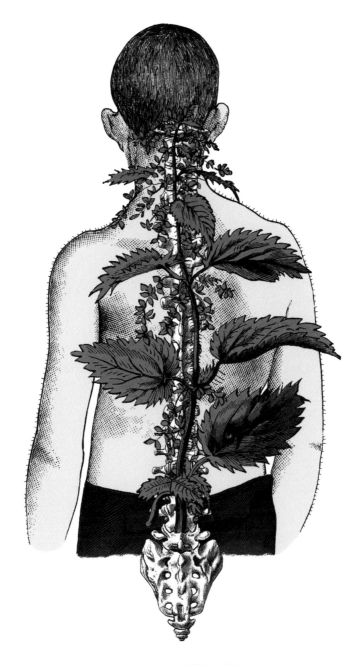

NETTLE • SKELETON

HOUSELEEK

Sempervivum tectorum

OTHER COMMON NAMES

common houseleek, plants of the housetops, hens and chicks, thunderbird,
thunder plant, thunder forever, roof foil, roof houseleek, welcome-home-husband-
however-drunk-you-be, earwort, homewort, Jupiter's eye, St Patrick's cabbage,
Aaron's rod, aye green, bullock's eye, Thor's beard, Jupiter's beard, bullock's
beard, devil's beard, Jove's beard, imbroke, poor Jan's leaf,
red-leaved houseleek, sengreen, live-forever

GIVEN TO HUMANKIND by the Greek god Zeus to protect houses from lightning and fire, it was not long before houseleek was being encouraged to grow on the roofs of ancient homes – and under the rule of the superstitious Roman emperor Charlemagne having such health and safety obligations forced on you by decree.

This hardy and succulent evergreen grows in mountainous regions of central Europe, and is commonly found on walls and buildings. The species name *tectorum* is translated as being 'of the roofs'.

Houseleek leaves, which come in multiple rosettes with occasional pink or yellow, star-shaped flowers, are harvested during summer. Studies show the leaves contain a juice (not unlike aloe vera; see page 142) that can be made into a poultice or ointment to tighten and soften skin, to soothe and cool burns, to heal minor wounds, insect bites and other skin problems from boils, warts, corns and sores to abscesses and nettle rashes.

Drinking tea prepared from the plant's leaves was once suggested for ulcer treatment, septic throats, bronchitis and mouth ailments, although chewing the occasional leaf is no longer recommended as an ease for toothache as it can induce vomiting.

Over the generations houseleek has picked up some interesting nicknames relating to its power to withstand thunder, as well as more impressionistic ones, like hens and chicks in recognition of the way the lateral rosettes of the leaves split from the mother plant to regenerate.

One name that cannot be ignored is welcome-home-husband-however-drunk-you-be, which some folklorists believe to be linked to an old culinary claim that meat spiced with houseleek increases male virility. Perhaps you will be better off sticking with houseleek as an aid for earache – a practice that comes with far more clinical credibility.

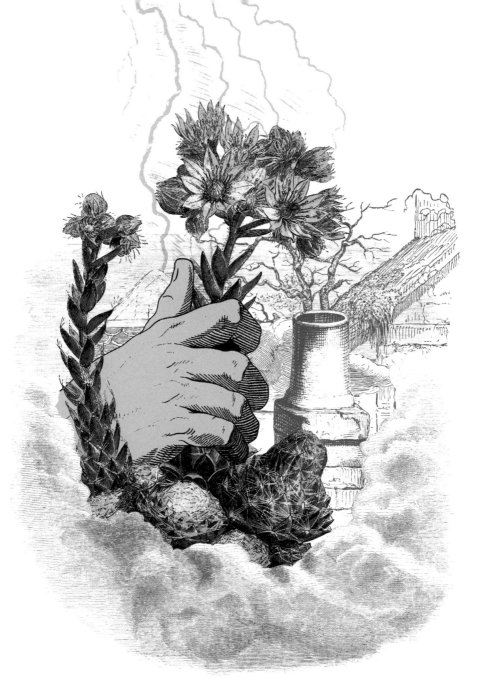

HOUSELEEK • SKELETON

CALENDULA

Calendula officinalis

OTHER COMMON NAMES
marigold, pot marigold, holigold, bride of Beth Sun, drunkard, husbandsman's dial,
marybud, margold, Mary gold, Mary gowles, golds, ruddies, summer bridge,
sun bride, Melvyn Mair, Jackanapes-on-horseback

THE SUN-LIKE blooms of this annual flower have been held sacred for centuries in various cultures, and it remains revered among herbalists the world over as a leading ingredient for skin lotions and ointments.

The antiseptic, antifungal and antibacterial qualities found in calendula flower heads are used in salves for skin complaints, wounds, burns and rashes, and can also be incorporated into poultices for stings. In fact, little of the plant need be wasted: sap from the stems can be used to treat warts, corns and calluses while eyewashes for conjunctivitis can be made from cold infusions of the whole plant.

This native of the Mediterranean has been prized for its positive associations with the radial power of the sun since ancient times. The common Western name of marigold is associated with Christianity and recurring symbolic themes related to the rising of the sun, rejuvenation and resurrection. Calendula is used to decorate the statues of Hindu deities, and is still incorporated into ceremonies and rituals in India and Arabia.

In addition to use in ceremonies and rituals, the Ancient Greeks and Egyptians enjoyed the petals as a saffron-like ingredient in cooking, and the Tudors are known to have coloured and flavoured cakes, soups and insipid stews with it – thus providing the nickname of pot marigold.

If you wish to keep evil away from your home you might want to hang a garland of calendula flowers over the doorway, or even scatter some of the petals under your pillow to make your dreams come true.

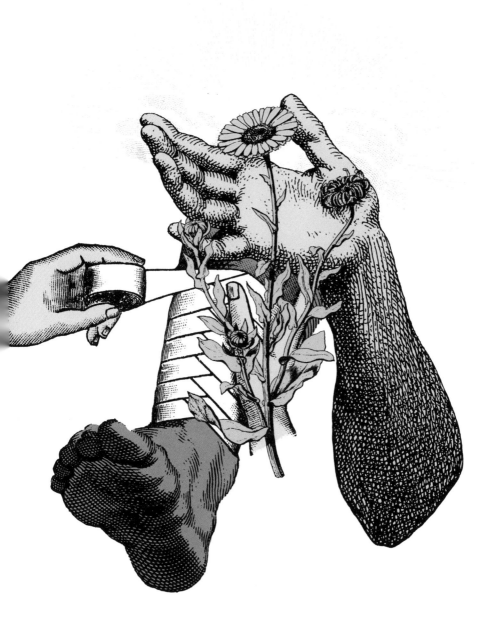

CALENDULA · SKELETON

LESSER CELANDINE

Ficaria verna

OTHER COMMON NAMES
pilewort, marsh pilewort, small celandine,
smallwort, brighteye, butter and cheese, scurvywort

LESSER CELANDINE WAS traditionally used as a reliever of haemorrhoids and ulcers, while medieval healers believed that simply carrying a handful of this invasive perennial around was enough to cure the piles of long-suffering patients.

The fact that the knobbly tubers of the plant resemble a particularly fearsome outbreak of such a painful ailment was grist to the mill for physicians who followed the *Doctrine of Signatures*, and it would subsequently go on to be commonly referred to as pilewort.

In the Western Isles of Scotland it was thought that the tubers resembled a cow's udder, so they hung them in byres to encourage high milk yields – earning the plant the nickname of butter and cheese. Providing an even more pleasing visual association for the tubers of this fan of European woodlands and hedgerows is the fact that its species name *ficaria* is derived from the Latin word for figs.

The German name for celandine is *Scharbockskraut*, which translates as 'scurvywort' in direct reference to the kind of ailment that the high levels of vitamin C contained in its glossy leaves might help to combat. Similarly the Russian name for the plant is *chistobel* ('clean body'), and in that country it is used in baths to help cure skin irritations such as dermatitis and rosacea.

Once seen as a 'visionary herb' that could increase psychic abilities, lesser celandine has also been imbibed in brews to induce pleasant dreams. Unfortunately, like its most common modern use as an ointment or suppository for treating haemorrhoids, there is little scientific evidence to support any such practices.

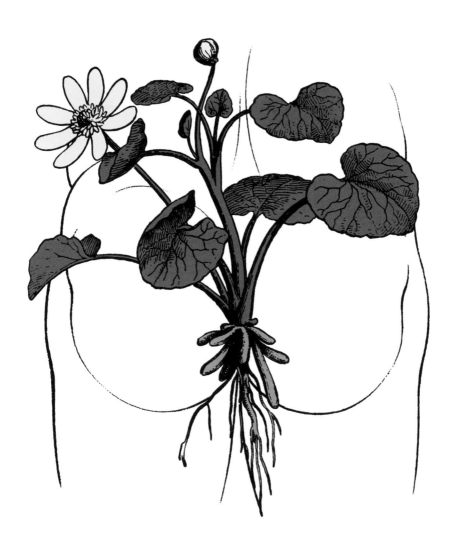

LESSER CELANDINE • SKELETON

OATS

Avena sativa

OTHER COMMON NAMES
groats, oatmeal, oat straw, wild oats, haver, common oat

IN SAMUEL JOHNSON's *Dictionary of the English Language* of 1755, the entry for oats reads: 'A grain which in England is generally given to horses, but in Scotland supports the people.' The Scottish riposte was: 'Aye, and that's why England has such fine horses, and Scotland such fine people.'

Still consumed as a way of maintaining muscle function during the training and exercise of both human and animal, this annual grass contains generous levels of vitamin B – a useful aid when it comes to building body tissue and stamina and supporting the immune system.

Oat grains and straw not only raise energy levels in a gentle way, but can act as a mild antidepressant to support the nervous system and can combat insomnia, nervous exhaustion and stress. In the 1800s doctors advocated a tea made of oat straw as a nerve tonic – a form of concoction that is still sold commercially today as a treatment for mild levels of anxiety.

Also said to have a positive impact on the thyroid, digestive system, blood-sugar levels and cigarette cravings, oats are usually eaten as a cereal or cholesterol-lowering bran. Less well known is the practice of stripping off and soaking in a strained decoction of oats as a soothing and cleansing benefit for those troubled by eczema and itchy skin complaints.

Recent studies show that consumption of oats can raise testosterone levels, which gives credence to the old farming tradition of giving the feed to stallions to encourage them to stud – as well as the old saying about young men wanting to 'sow their wild oats'.

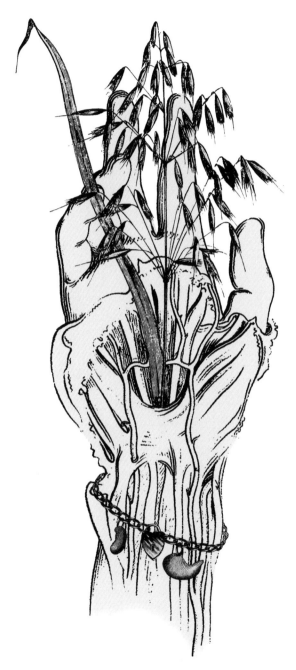

OATS • SKELETON

WITCH HAZEL

Hamamelis virginiana

OTHER COMMON NAMES
Virginian witch hazel, American witch hazel, snapping hazel nut, spotted alder,
striped alder, winterbloom, snapping hazelnut, tobacco weed

B EING ONE OF the most popular natural ingredients in the world
of skincare, from the fight against problematic medical conditions to cosmetic concerns, witch hazel is likely to be in the mix.

The key to the appeal of this woodland shrub or small tree is the tannins in its leaves and bark, which create a protective and astringent covering on skin abrasions – increasing resistance to inflammation, promoting rejuvenation in blood vessels and preventing infection.

Long since proven to be of value in the treatment of burns, scalds, insect bites and inflammatory conditions such as acne and eczema, witch hazel has also become a valued ingredient in cleansing, toning and anti-ageing products. Oil extracted from the bark of the plant is generally distilled for such items and is sometimes utilized in eyewashes as well as in salves for varicose veins, haemorrhoids and bruises.

Indigenous to North America but now cultivated in Europe, the leaves of witch hazel are gathered and dried in summer and the bark is harvested in autumn.

Native Americans fashioned poultices from soaked bark to treat tumours and inflammations (particularly in eyes) and used the leaves to address internal haemorrhaging and heavy menstrual bleeding.

In a practice known as 'witching a well', the eighteenth-century European colonizers of North America made use of the pliable nature of the species as a dowsing rod in their search for suitable new watering holes. It is thought that the first part of its common name is derived from the word *wych* or *wice*, which is the Anglo-Saxon term for 'bend'. These colonizers would have used common hazel (*Corylus avellana*) for dowsing rods in their original countries in Europe, so it appears they merged the name of their new tool with their old one to come up with the new moniker of witch hazel.

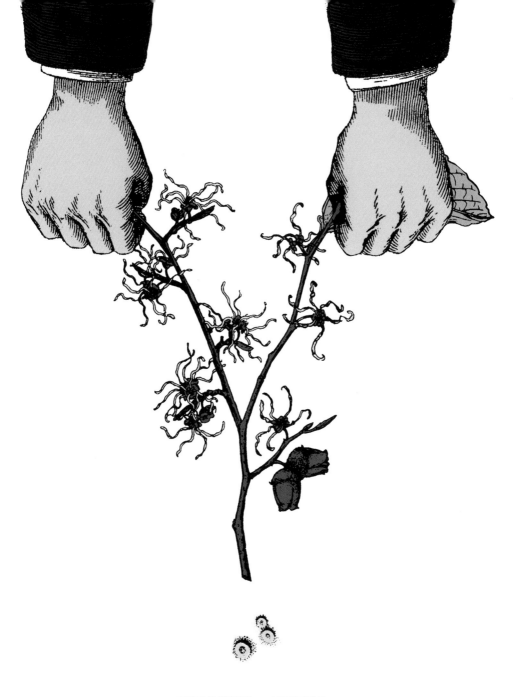

WITCH HAZEL • SKELETON

WINTERGREEN

Gaultheria procumbens

OTHER COMMON NAMES
boxberry, Canada tea, canterberry, checkerberry, chickenberry,
creeping wintergreen, deerberry, drunkards, gingerberry, ground berry,
ground tea, grouseberry, hillberry, mountain tea, squaw vine,
star berry, spiceberry, spicy wintergreen, teaberry

DURING THE AMERICAN War of Independence in the eighteenth century, the leaves of this low-lying shrub were used as a replacement for the tea leaves that had traditionally been imported from the colonies by the British. In doing so the new republicans were harking back to a far older tradition.

Native Americans and Canadians had drunk tea-like infusions of wintergreen for generations as a treatment for back pain, rheumatism, fever, headaches, sore throats and to soothe painful joints.

A native of central and eastern North America, this small shrub favours woodland and exposed mountainous areas and has leathery, oval leaves, small white and pink flowers, and brilliant red fruit. Its ripe berries taste like an uncomfortably strong and fragrant peppermint.

Herbalists gather wintergreen leaves and berries in summer. When crushed they emit a camphor-like smell that is used as a flavouring that will be familiar to those who use Germoline ointment or Euthymol toothpaste, or who drink certain root beers.

Containing pain-relieving salicylic acid, which is a strong anti-inflammatory and antiseptic present in aspirin, wintergreen has been used for relieving arthritic problems. When taken as a tea it can soothe the digestive system and relieve flatulence and colic, while essential oils, balms or ointments are popular with sportsmen suffering from the kind of muscular pains connected to intense physical workouts, such as sprains, cramps, stretched muscles, ligaments and backaches.

Often sold as a decorative seasonal pot plant in European supermarkets and garden centres, it is easy to forget that this evergreen was once the toast of kings – its botanical name *Gaultheria* coming from Jean-François Gaulthier, an eighteenth-century surgeon and botanist to the king of France, Louis XV, who 'discovered' the plant on a posting to Quebec.

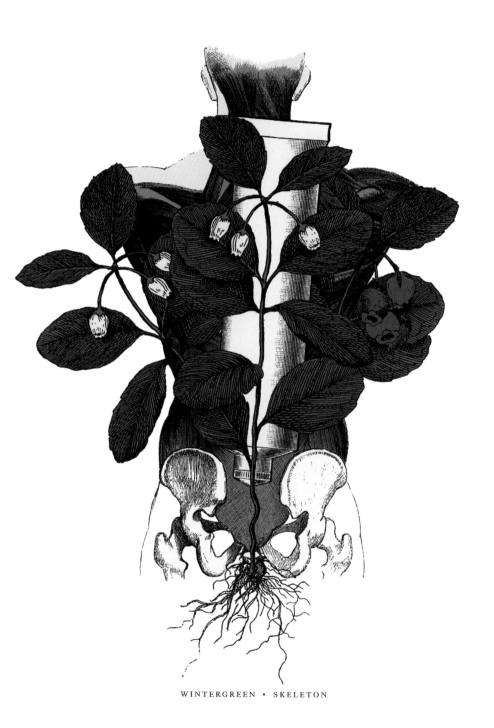

WINTERGREEN · SKELETON

ARNICA

Arnica montana

OTHER COMMON NAMES
mountain arnica, mountain daisy, mountain tobacco,
medicinal leopard's bane, mountain alkanet

THIS TOUGH PERENNIAL grows in alpine woods and pastures, and for centuries has been held in high esteem as an anti-inflammatory by European herbalists.

Best known as an effective ointment and compress for bruises, sprains and muscle pain, arnica improves the local blood supply to damaged areas and can accelerate healing. A stimulant of circulation, it might be of particular value to those suffering from angina and weak or failing hearts and could also be used to treat rheumatic pain and chilblains.

The leaves and roots of the plant have traditionally been dried and smoked as a popular herbal tobacco, and there are historic references (which come without any modern scientific provenance) to its addition as a stimulant for hair growth and the treatment of epilepsy and seasickness.

Commonly found growing in Europe, the flowers of the plant are harvested in summer and the roots in autumn.

Arnica should not be applied to broken skin as it can cause rashes and irritation, and you might also want to think twice about handling it if you do not have a handkerchief to hand – just one sniff of arnica will make most people sneeze – its name being said to be derived from the Greek word *ptarmikos* ('sneezing').

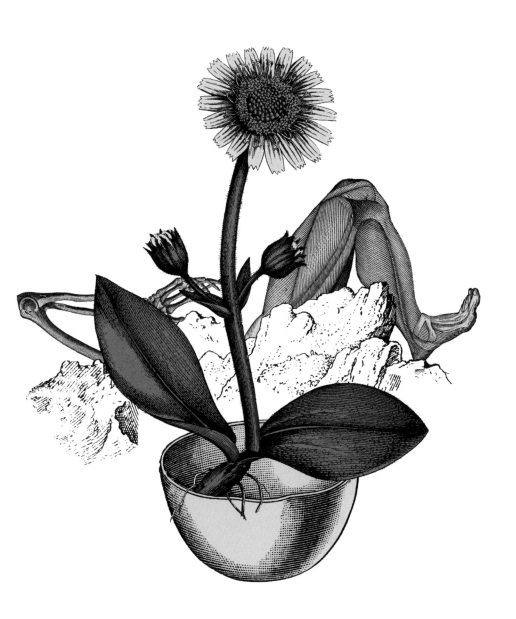

ARNICA • SKELETON

SELFHEAL

Prunella vulgaris

OTHER COMMON NAMES

carpenter's herb, heal-all, all-heal, blue curls, heart-of-the-earth, prunella, brunella,
carpenter weed, hook heal, slough heal, blue Lucy, brownwort, brunel,
caravaun bog, carpenter grass, carpenter's square, herb carpenter,
Hercules's all-heal, hookweed, proud carpenter, sickle-heal,
sicklewort, slough heal, square stem, thimble flower

CHINESE PHYSICIANS HAVE drawn on the anti-inflammatory properties of this creeping perennial for thousands of years, while tradesmen and labourers of all cultures have long drawn on its healing powers as a balm for work-related injuries.

The hook-like appearance of the upper lip of each of the plant's flowers was most important in the formalization of its role in Western medicine when it appeared in the *Doctrine of Signatures* in the sixteenth century – the hook being seen as symbolic of the fact that the use of billhooks and sickles often resulted in wounds during agricultural cultivation.

This plant, from the northern hemisphere, is best harvested when in bloom during the summer months. It thrives by waysides, meadows and on farmland – often growing close to where agricultural accidents took place, providing further evidence for the physicians that it was a wound-healer worthy of the title selfheal. Later pseudonyms such as sicklewort, hookweed and carpenter grass were tied to the same theme of agricultural or artisan injury.

The medical value that healers of the period placed on links between human ailments and the appearance of plants was brought to bear twice over with selfheal – courtesy of the claim that the shape of a throat could be seen within the flower spike's violet and pink blooms. Not unlike the Ancient Greek physicians before them, sixteenth-century healers saw the plant once again being used to treat diseases of the throat, like quinsy and diphtheria, as well as for brews to help with sore throats and tonsilitis.

Selfheal continues to be used by modern herbalists to staunch bleeding and heal wounds and to soothe burns and bruises, as well as being prescribed as a gargle for sore throats and inflammation in the mouth. It appears that the healers of the Early Modern period thankfully got this one right.

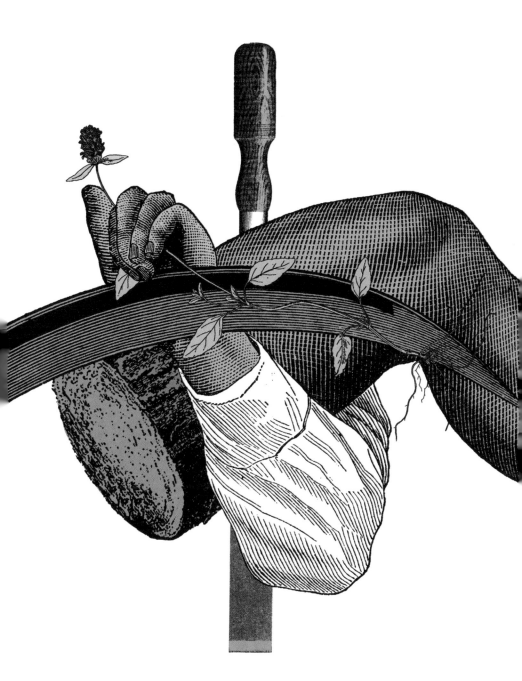

SELFHEAL • SKELETON

WILLOW

Salix alba

OTHER COMMON NAMES
European willow, white willow, Huntingdon willow,
swallow-tailed willow

ANCIENT EGYPTIAN, GREEK, Sumerian and Assyrian medical texts all feature the dried, rough, grey bark of the willow tree as a remedy for aches, pains and fevers – and a line might well be drawn from them to the arrival of aspirin in 1899.

The English clergyman and naturalist Edward Stone is said to have set the scientific process in motion for the birth of aspirin when he began trials into the health benefits of dried willow bark in the 1750s. Inspired by his work, a new breed of European chemists separated the most active ingredient of the bark (salicylic acid) from its natural source, and this would go on to become the key ingredient of the new 'wonder drug' created by German scientists.

Modern clinical trials have shown that high-strength doses of willow bark can provide a successful alternative to anti-inflammatory medicines, particularly in relation to quality pain relief from osteoarthritis, lower back pain and painful discomfort in joints such as knees and hips. The salicylic acid found within the tree causes few side effects when taken in more natural forms and is now being widely researched as an alternative to traditional, aspirin-based anti-inflammatories, such as ibuprofen, which some people cannot take because of other underlying conditions that it inflames.

Described as a 'cooling' herb, herbalists believe extracts of willow can also reduce headaches, sweats and fevers, as well as help control menopausal symptoms such as hot flushes and night sweats.

This large tree is native to much of Europe and can grow up to 25m (82 ft) tall. It thrives in damp conditions, such as riverbanks, and is sometimes referred to as white willow because the undersides of its leaves are of a whitish hue.

There are many different varieties of willow, and artisans value it as much as healers for being a tough and durable wood that is light and pliable and easy to work with. No wonder the gift of willow on a May morning was deemed lucky.

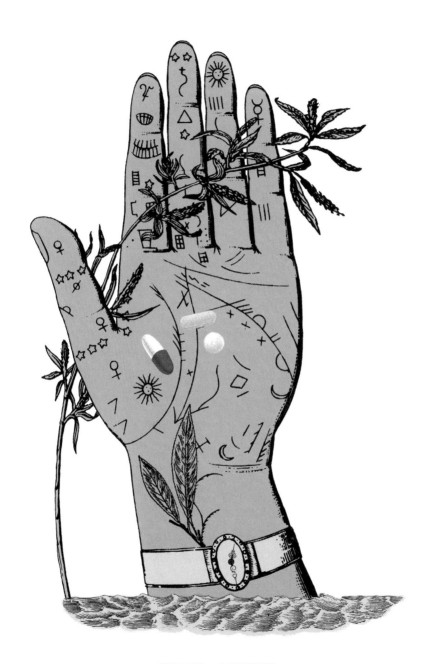

WILLOW • SKELETON

HORSETAIL

Equisetum arvense

OTHER COMMON NAMES
bottlebrush, scouring rush, field horsetail, common horsetail, giant horsetail,
shave grass, paddock pipes, Dutch rushes, pewterwort

THIS PRIMITIVE PLANT with no direct affinity to any of its more modern counterparts is descended from a super-sized ancestor that could grow up to 30m (100ft) tall and which was itself a descendant of the Palaeozoic era of more than 300 million years ago.

Long considered a wound-healing herb, horsetail (which now grows to around 35cm/14in) contains large amounts of silicic acid, silicates and alkaloids (including nicotine) that support the regeneration of connective tissues and the clotting of blood.

Native to Europe, North Asia and the Americas, the plant prefers damp soil. The sterile, needle-like stems, which can be surprisingly fragile to pick, are carefully harvested and dried in summer. In Europe, young stems of the earlier and larger species of the plant were eaten and dressed like asparagus or fried with flour and butter, and poorer Romans ate them as a vegetable. While Western diners may no longer view them as being particularly nutritious or palatable, the shoots are still a feature of numerous Korean dishes.

Modern herbalists use horsetail to heal wounds and stop nosebleeds, as well as a support to the urinary system in cases of cystitis, urethritis and prostate disease. Horsetail might also feature as a treatment for kidney and bladder problems, haemorrhaging ulcers, arthritis and rheumatism and chest complaints such as emphysema.

The high silica content of horsetail makes the plant quite abrasive to the touch, and it was used by dairymaids to clean milk pails (hence the common name scouring brush), to polish metal and wood and to smooth rough surfaces (shavegrass) and as a key component of sweeping brushes (bottlebrush).

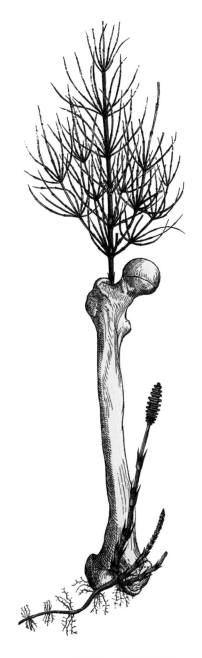

HORSETAIL • SKELETON

INDEX

ACKNOWLEDGEMENTS

WITH MANY THANKS to Martin Purdy for enlivening the book by turning my notes into prose. Alice Graham, the commissioning editor, for stumbling across my work and making the idea evolve into this book. The Frances Lincoln team, notably Bella Skertchly, Paileen Currie and Isabel Eeles for their stoic support and involvement in the project. Infinitely grateful to Christian Brett – my partner, pacemaker, backbone and in-house typesetter. My family Julian and Mary and Ben Smith, Allen and Pauline and Charlotte Brett, for their support and encouragement throughout. Graham Moss and Kathy Whalen for an endless source of knowledge, laughter, and inspiration that contributed towards the evolution of this book. Penny Rimbaud, Gee Vaucher and Bron Jones for the energy, imagination, nourishment that inspired the original series of illustrations. Penny Waters for introducing and instilling an addiction to worts. Dominique Van Cappellen, Sue Shaw, Alessandra Mostyn for being great cheerleaders and facilitators of this series. Tom Hodgkinson and Victoria Hull for their support and busyness. John Mitchinson for the sound advice. My allotment society and neighbours for overlooking my weeds and strange plant growing habits this last year. And to friends and family for their support throughout the strange pandemic years from which this book was born.

Thanks also to: The Wellcome Collection, Kew Gardens, Chelsea Physic Garden and the RHS for being a font of knowledge and inspiration throughout my self-taught meanderings. To Monty Don, James Wong, Gertrude Jekyll, Maud Grieve, John Gerard, Nicholas Culpeper, Pedanius Dioscorides and all the plants-people throughout history, for being bold enough to put down on paper simply because you believe, and have found, and say it is so. To all the medical and botanical illustrators from centuries ago who've left legacies on which I have fed and stolen. To the generations of scientists and medical researchers and practitioners who keep an open mind to revisiting old and new knowledge.

– Alice Smith

ABOUT THE AUTHORS

ALICE SMITH is an artist, freelance illustrator and designer based in Lancashire, UK. She is the art director for *Idler* magazine and is the co-founder of Bracketpress, which publishes work by an eclectic group of maverick writers and musicians. Her work has been exhibited at various venues in the UK, USA and in Europe, and Alice regularly exhibits and sells her work at print fairs in the UK.

MARTIN PURDY is a freelance writer, historian, Doctor of Philosophy and a member of the folk song and storytelling collective Harp & a Monkey. His published works include *Doing Our Bit* and *The Gallipoli Oak*, and research titles for the BBC's *Who Do You Think You Are?* franchise.

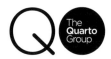

First published in 2022 by Frances Lincoln,
an imprint of The Quarto Group.
The Old Brewery, 6 Blundell Street, London N7 9BH
www.quarto.com

A catalogue record for this book is available
from the British Library.

ISBN 978-0-7112-6633-9

EBOOK ISBN 978-0-7112-6634-6

10 9 8 7 6 5 4 3 2 1

Printed in China

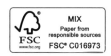